BASIC CONCEPTS IN
IMMUNOLOGY

Notice

Medicine is an ever-changing science. As new research and clinical experience broaden our knowledge, changes in treatment and drug therapy are required. The author and the publisher of this work have checked with sources believed to be reliable in their efforts to provide information that is complete and generally in accord with the standards accepted at the time of publication. However, in view of the possibility of human error or changes in medical sciences, neither the author nor the publisher nor any other party who has been involved in the preparation or publication of this work warrants that the information contained herein is in every respect accurate or complete, and they are not responsible for any errors or omissions or for the results obtained from use of such information. Readers are encouraged to confirm the information contained herein with other sources. For example and in particular, readers are advised to check the product information sheet included in the package of each drug they plan to administer to be certain that the information contained in this book is accurate and that changes have not been made in the recommended dose or in the contraindications for administration. This recommendation is of particular importance in connection with new or infrequently used drugs.

BASIC CONCEPTS IN
IMMUNOLOGY

A STUDENT'S SURVIVAL GUIDE

JOHN CLANCY, Jr., Ph.D.

Professor and Chair
of
Cell Biology, Neurobiology and Anatomy
Loyola University Medical Center
Maywood, Illinois

Series Editor
Hiram F. Gilbert, Ph.D.

The McGraw-Hill Companies
Health Professions Division

New York   St. Louis   San Francisco
Auckland   Bogota   Caracus   Lisbon   London   Madrid
Mexico City   Milan   Montreal   New Delhi   Paris   San Juan
Singapore   Sydney   Tokyo   Toronto

McGraw-Hill Higher Education ℠

A Division of The McGraw-Hill Companies

BASIC CONCEPTS IN IMMUNOLOGY:
A STUDENT'S SURVIVAL GUIDE

34567890 QSR/QSR 09876543

ISBN: 0-07-011371-8

This book was set in Times Roman by Better Graphics, Inc. The editors were James Morgan and Pamela Touboul; the series editor was Hiram F. Gilbert, Ph.D.; the production supervisor was Richard Ruzycka; the project manager was Hockett Editorial Service; the cover designer was Marsha Cohen; the cover illustrator was Phong Le, Ph.D.

Quebecor World Dubuque was printer and binder.

This book is printed on acid-free paper.

Cover: In order for most adaptive immune responses to be initiated, antigenic peptide must be presented by an antigen presenting cell (APC) in the context of its own MHC-II to the CD3-TCR complex of a CD4 Th cell. Chapter 8 of this book will help you understand the mechanisms and consequences of this interaction.

Library of Congress Cataloging-in-Publication Data

Basic concepts on immunology : a student's survival guide / [edited by] John Clancy, Jr.
   p.   cm.
  Includes index.
  ISBN 0-07-011371-8
  1. Immunology. 2. Immunity. I. Clancy, John, 1943–   .
  [DNLM: 1. Immunity—physiology. 2. Immunologic Diseases—immunology. 3. Immune System—physiology. QW 540 B311 1998]
QR181.B29   1998
616.07′9   cc21
DNLM/DLC
for Library of Congress   97-25668

· C O N T E N T S ·

CHAPTER 9   HUMORAL IMMUNITY   91

CHAPTER 10   INFLAMMATION   101

CHAPTER 11   ANATOMICAL LOCATION OF
   IMMUNE RESPONSES   111

CHAPTER 12   IMMEDIATE HYPERSENSITIVITY   117

CHAPTER 13   DELAYED TYPE HYPERSENSITIVITY (DTH)

CHAPTER 14   COMPLEMENT VERSUS CELL-MEDIATED LYSIS

CHAPTER 15   MICROBIAL IMMUNITY AND IMMUNOPARASITOLOGY

CHAPTER 16   AUTOIMMUNITY

· C O N T R I B U T O R S ·

JOHN CLANCY, Jr., Ph.D.
Professor and Chair of Cell Biology, Neurobiology and Anatomy

ELIZABETH J. KOVACS, Ph.D.
Associate Professor of Cell Biology, Neurobiology and Anatomy

PHONG T. LE, Ph.D.
Associate Professor of Cell Biology, Neurobiology and Anatomy

LINDA A. PICCININI, Ph.D.
Assistant Professor of Cell Biology, Neurobiology and Anatomy

JOHN A. ROBINSON, M.D.
Professor of Medicine and Microbiology and Immunology
Associate Dean of Research

VIRGINIA M. SANDERS, Ph.D.
Assistant Professor of Cell Biology, Neurobiology and Anatomy
and Microbiology and Immunology

PAMELA L. WITTE, Ph.D.
Associate Professor of Cell Biology, Neurobiology and Anatomy
and Microbiology and Immunology

· P R E F A C E ·

Basic Concepts in Immunology: A Student's Survival Guide is not a conventional textbook or review book. It is designed to explain the important concepts of immunology in a clear and concise manner.

There are many comprehensive texts of immunology that do an excellent job in presenting numerous facts in this rapidly developing and ever-changing field. We have attempted to synthesize these facts into clear explanatory presentations of what we and our students feel are the most challenging areas of immunology. Each of the 18 chapters represents the main areas of focus that we and our students feel are necessary to master for an understanding of the basic concepts in immunology. Below each chapter title are the main subjects or simplest concepts found in that chapter. These subjects are clearly defined in a stepwise fashion. Summary diagrams and tables are used where appropriate. Extensive references to previous and following chapters are used throughout; however, each chapter stands on its own in explaining the topic. All the CD antigens used in the book are concisely summarized in Appendix 1, and the cytokines in Appendix 2. The main terms used in the book are briefly defined in the Glossary.

We hope that this book will help not only the beginning, but also the advanced student, to integrate some of the basic areas in this rapidly growing and fascinating field.

ACKNOWLEDGMENTS

I would like to give a very special thanks to my wife and best friend, Kathy, for her continued support and encouragement. Also, my mother Katherine, for teaching me how and what to write.

The contributors and I would like to thank Gail Gavert and Jim Morgan at McGraw-Hill Health Professions Division for asking us to write this book, as well as for their encouragement. We would also like to thank Rachel Youngman of Hockett Editorial Service for her editorial skills and Joanna Goral for critically reading the manuscript.

In addition, I would like to thank Christine Creadon for translating many of our wishes into figures and Ginny Hayes for typing and formatting many of the chapters.

John Clancy, Jr.

BASIC CONCEPTS IN
IMMUNOLOGY

DEFINITION OF GENERAL ASPECTS OF IMMUNE RESPONSES

·

- **Innate Immunity**
- **Adaptive (Acquired) Immunity**
- **Clonal Selection**
- **Humoral and Cellular Immunity**

· · · · · · · · · · · ·

The innate and adaptive immune systems protect us from potentially infectious agents (viruses, bacteria, etc.) that have gained access to our body through the skin or the lining of our internal organs. Such systems have evolved to protect us from not only intracellular (viruses, some smaller parasites, some bacteria) and from extracellular (most bacteria, large parasites) pathogens and allergens (animal hair, pollen, chemicals) but also from ourselves in potentially uncontrolled growth such as malignancy or autoimmune diseases.

INNATE IMMUNITY

Innate immunity is a nonspectific cellular and humoral response that operates as the first line of defense against pathogens. Extracellular pathogens are immediately taken up and degraded by neutrophils and mononuclear phagocytes. Large parasites are killed by eosinophils. Natural killer lymphocytes kill some tumor and virally infected cells. Preexisting soluble mediators of innate immunity are natural antibodies and serum complement components, which can also attach to the cell membranes of many pathogens.

The main characteristics and components of innate immunity occur in the inflammatory response discussed in Chap. 10. If an organism enters the body by breaking through the barriers of the skin or mucosa lining the inner surfaces of the body, it comes in contact with phagocytic (neutrophils, eosinophils, monocytes/macrophages) and/or natural killer cells as well as the complement system. Complement consists of over 20 proteins, all of which interact in a cascade fashion to attract phagocytic cells (chemotaxis), coat bacteria (opsonize) so that phagocytic cells recognize and then engulf them, and interact with antibody to lyse the cell membrane of the invading organism (Chap. 14). Thus, the main mediators of innate immunity are lysosomal enzymes and interferons as well as other cytokines, complement proteins, and acute phase proteins (Table 1-1).

It should be noted that innate host defenses are found in all multicellular organisms, most of which do not have an adaptive immune system. However, in multicellular organisms with an adaptive system, many of the mediators of innate immunity can recruit adaptive immune cells.

ADAPTIVE (ACQUIRED) IMMUNITY

Adaptive immunity is a highly specific, inducible, discriminatory, and unforgetting T lymphocyte-dependent response. Normal adaptive responses operate under *major histocompatibility complex (MHC) restriction.*

In order to handle certain pathogens, multicellular organisms have developed a group of largely circulating cells with very specific receptors for immunogenic peptide fragments of both intracellular and extracellular pathogens. When these receptors are activated, the cells can secrete various soluble mediators that

TABLE 1-1
DIFFERENCES BETWEEN INNATE AND ADAPTIVE IMMUNITY

	REPEATED EXPOSURE	MEMORY	EFFECTORS	MOLECULES
Innate	Same intensity against all antigens	No	Neutrophils, macrophages, eosinophils, NK cells	Complement lysosomal enzymes, acute phase proteins, interferons
Adaptive	More rapid and intense (memory)	Yes	T and B lymphocytes	Cytokines, antibodies

attack pathogens directly (antibodies, perforin granules, etc.) or stimulate other cells (cytokines) to do so. This army of circulating cells will be discussed in more detail in Chap. 2 but generally involve B and T lymphocytes and various antigen-presenting cells (monocytes, macrophages, and dendritic cells). Antigen-presenting cells either process or present already processed antigenic peptides to surface immunoglobin receptors on B cells and immunoglobin-like receptors of T cells. While surface immunoglobin on B cells can directly respond to an immunogenic piece (epitope) of a pathogen, in order to develop into mature plasma cells, they usually require some help in the form of cytokines from T cells (Fig. 1-1).

Thus, T cells are central to an adaptive immune response. Helper T (Th) cells not only help B cells become plasma cells, they can also help cytotoxic T cells develop as well as increase macrophage activity. However, in contrast to B cells, the receptors on the surface of T cells can only recognize processed antigenic epitopes presented to them in the context of surface MHC. The ability

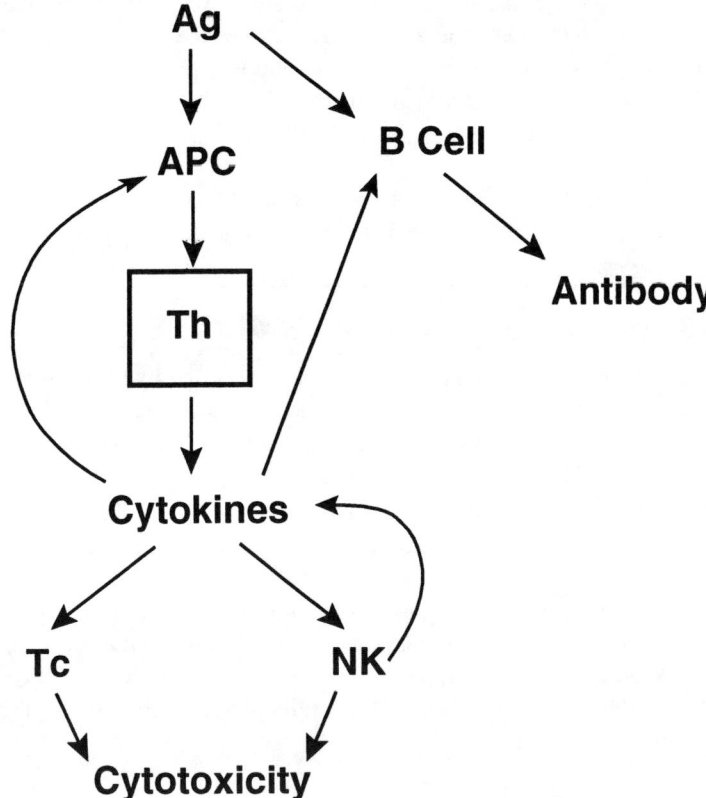

Figure 1-1
Th cells central to adaptive immune response.

of T cells to see only foreign antigen in the context of self MHC is called *MHC restriction* and is a critical safeguard for the adaptive immune system to only eliminate pathogens and not normal cells. The MHC will be discussed in detail in Chap. 6.

Finally, an adaptive immune response displays a high degree of memory. Even though you will learn in Chaps. 2, 4, and 5 that T and B cells develop with their appropriate receptors for a cognate antigen's epitope without ever seeing that antigen before, once encountering that antigen and generating a full immune response to it, they will remember such a first encounter. Thus, when these memory T and B cells encounter that same antigen again their response to that antigen is much faster and more robust.

CLONAL SELECTION

When antigen binds to either surface immunoglobulin on B cells or its specific receptor on T cells, these cells are induced to proliferate rapidly. Thus, antigen selects and generates specific clones that bind and respond to it. This process is called *clonal selection* and is an extremely important part of the adaptive immune response (Fig. 1-2).

The nature of the specific receptors on B and T cells will be discussed in Chaps. 4 and 5 as well as differences between naive and memory cells.

HUMORAL AND CELLULAR IMMUNITY

Humoral immunity is mediated by the antibody secreted by terminally differentiated B cells, the plasma cells. *Cell-mediated immunity* involves T cells that recognize antigen in an MHC-restricted fashion and either secrete cytokines (Th cells) or become cytotoxic cells (Tc cells), which kill virus-infected cells or abnormal host cells.

It should be realized that in many cases a normal humoral response will not proceed unless there is also a companion Th cell response; this is because Th cells secrete various cytokines (Appendix 2) that are necessary for full B cell maturation and antibody class switching. The details of such a response will be discussed in Chaps. 9 and 11.

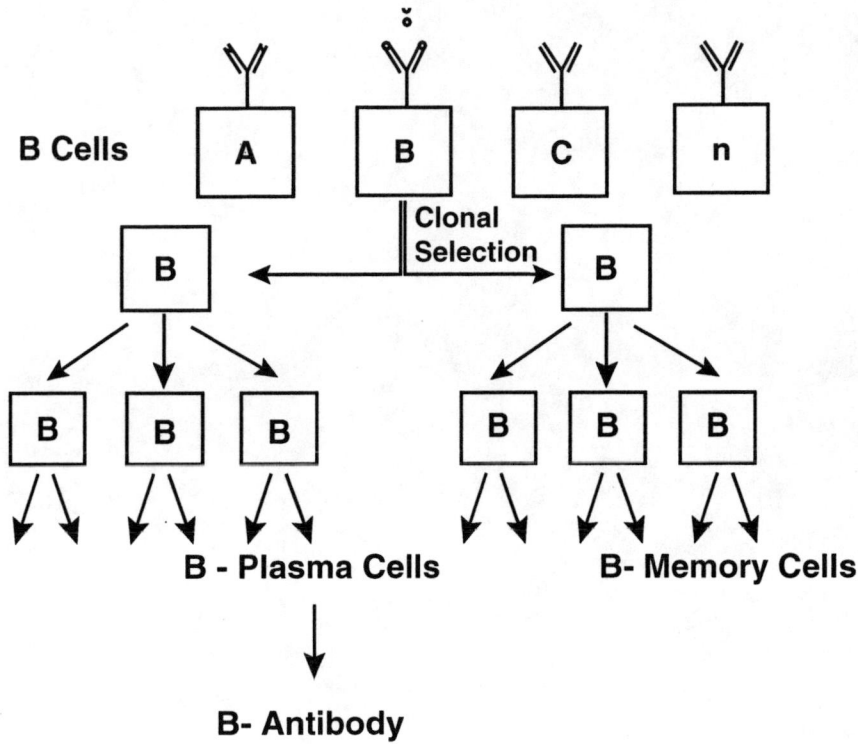

Figure 1-2
Clonal selection.

· C H A P T E R · 2 ·

ORIGIN, DESTINATION, AND STRUCTURE OF CELLS AND TISSUES OF THE IMMUNE SYSTEM

·

- **Bone Marrow**
- **Stem Cells**
- **Erythropoiesis**
- **Granulocytopoiesis**

    Eosinophils

    Basophils

    Neutrophils

- **Lymphopoiesis**
- **Natural Killer Cells**
- **Monocytes**
- **Dendritic Cells**
- **Thymus**
- **Lymph Nodes**
- **Spleen**
- **Mucosal Associated Lymphoid Tissue (MALT)**
- **Circulation and Recirculation**

BONE MARROW

The bone marrow constitutes almost 5% of total body weight and is responsible for the formation of all blood cells (*hemopoiesis*) in adults. It also provides a microenvironment necessary for B lymphocyte maturation and formation of pre-T cells (*lymphopoiesis*).

STEM CELLS

All of these cells originate from undifferentiated pluripotential hemopoietic *stem cells* (PHSC), which can be found first in the mammalian embryo within the liver then spleen. SCs are pluripotential CD34+ and represent less than 0.1% of all cells in adult marrow. SCs have limited proliferative capacity and exhibit the potential to differentiate into all cells of the myeloid (erythrocytes, granulocytes, monocytes, and platelets) or lymphoid (T and B cells) lineage. When SCs divide, the two *daughter cells* (*DCs*) can either continue as SCs or proceed into any of the differentiation pathways (Fig. 2-1).

If a DC proceeds into the differentiation pathway, it becomes a dividing multipotential colony forming unit-spleen (CFU-S) or CFU-lymphoid (CFU-Ly) progenitor cell and then a progressively maturing unipotential precursor cell for any of the mature cells of peripheral blood. The precursor cell gradually loses its ability to self-renew and then divide as it approaches its mature phenotype. SCs not only depend on a specific microenvironment for their maturation, they also depend on numerous glycoprotein growth factors that act at different stages to control the cell type as well as rate of cell formation. Some of these growth factors such as stem cell factor (SCF) and interleukin (IL)-7 are secreted by marrow stromal cells, but most others are produced elsewhere and transported to the marrow by the blood stream (endocrine).

ERYTHROPOIESIS

Erythropoiesis occurs when a CFU-S cell gives rise to burst-forming units-erythrocyte (BFU-E) and then colony-forming units-erythrocyte (CFU-E) all under the influence of *erythropoietin* (*EPO*) from the kidney cortex as well as IL-3 and granulocyte-macrophage colony-stimulating factor (GM-CSF) (Appendix 2).

CFU-E form the precursor of erythrocytes, the proerythroblast. Under normal conditions, 2.5×10^{11} erythrocytes are produced each day. Proerythroblast $\to$ basophilic erythroblast $\to$ polychromatophilic erythroblast $\to$ orthochromatophilic erythroblast $\to$ reticulocyte $\to$ erythrocyte is the sequence of events in maturation. During this sequence, the nucleus is condensed and then lost as the cell becomes 6-7μ. These maturation events occur around macrophages, which phagocytose the extruded nuclei as well as provide some growth factors.

GRANULOCYTOPOIESIS

Granulocytopoiesis is the generation of three types of granulocytes (neutrophils, eosinophils, basophils) from CFU-S. Mature cells are named because of staining of their specific granules. All derive from CFU-S $\to$ CFU-Eo, $-$BASO or CFU-NM $\to$ CFU-N $\to$ myeloblast $\to$ promyelocyte $\to$ myelocyte $\to$ metamyelocyte $\to$ Stab $\to$ mature cell (Fig. 2-1).

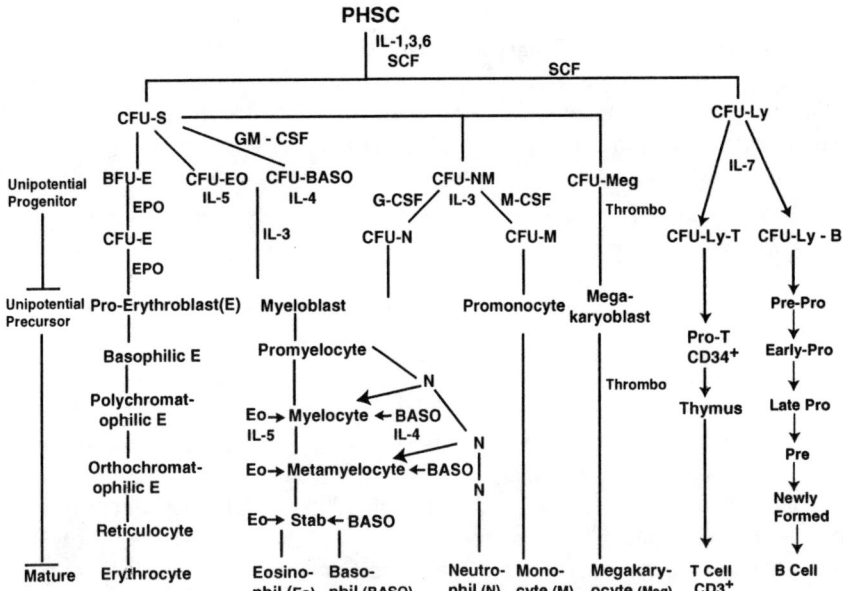

Figure 2-1
Cells and growth factors in hemopoiesis.

Eosinophils

Eosinophils require GM-CSF, IL-3, and IL-5 for their maturation. They represent 2 to 4% of peripheral blood white cells. Their specific granules contain a number of factors including histaminase, acid phosphatase, and major basic protein. They are important in destroying parasites, phagocytosing antigen-antibody complexes, and combating histamine levels during allergic reactions.

Basophils

Basophils require GM-CSF, IL-3, and IL-4 for their maturation. They represent <1% of peripheral blood white cells. Their specific granules contain histamine, heparin, and chemotactic factors for eosinophils and neutrophils. They are similar to mast cells in that they participate in IgE-mediated immediate hypersensitivity responses (Chap. 12).

Neutrophils

Neutrophils require GM-CSF, IL-3, and granulocyte colony-stimulating factor (G-CSF) for their maturation. Unlike eosinophils and basophils, the CFU-S gives rise to a CFU-NM cell, which, depending on the level of granulocyte or macrophage colony-stimulating factor in the environment, can differentiate into a CFU-Neut or CFU-M cell. Sixty to 70% of all white cells are neutrophils. Their specific granules contain alkaline phosphatase, lysozyme, lactoferrin, phagocytin, and type IV collagenase. They are the earliest phagocytic cells to appear in a bacterial infection and are a prominent constituent of pus.

LYMPHOPOIESIS

Lymphopoiesis is the ability of CFU-Ly to form either CFU-LyB or CFU-LyT in the bone marrow.

CFU-LyB cells develop in the presence of IL-7 and IL-3 in the marrow to immunocompetent *B cells* with sIgM (Chap. 4). Further maturation of these cells occurs in germinal centers of secondary lymphoid tissue. CFU-Ly T cells become *pre-T cells*, which leave the bone marrow and find their way to the subcapsular area of the thymic cortex where they proliferate and mature in the deeper thymic cortex into either $CD3^+4^+$ or $CD3^+8^+$ cells (Chap. 5). Thus, the bone marrow and thymus are considered primary lymphoid tissue, and lymph nodes, spleen, gut-associated lymphoid tissue, etc. are considered secondary lymphoid tissue.

NATURAL KILLER CELLS

Natural killer (NK) cells also develop within the marrow and then are found in peripheral blood, liver sinusoids (pit cells), and spleen sinusoids but not thoracic duct lymph. NK cells appear early in bacterial infections, can secrete interferon-γ, and spontaneously kill some viral infected cells and tumor cells. They respond to IL-2 and develop independently of the thymus.

MONOCYTES

Monocytes develop from CFU-M progenitors under the influence of GM-CSF, IL-3, and G-CSF. They represent 3 to 8% of leukocytes in peripheral blood.

Monocytes have numerous azurophilic granules (lysosomes) in their cytoplasm and can readily leave the circulation to give rise to macrophages within almost every organ. They are thus the source of the *mononuclear phagocytic system* throughout the body. They are even more phagocytic than neutrophils or eosinophils in that they can degrade larger bacteria within phagosomes via the formation of hydrogen peroxide, hypochlorous acid, and superoxide. They can also fuse to form foreign body giant cells in response to a large antigenic load. Macrophages express class II major histocompatibility complex and can function as antigen-processing and -presenting cells (Chap. 7). They secrete the proinflammatory cytokines IL-1, IL-6, and tumor necrosis factor α (TNFα) upon activation (Chap. 15).

DENDRITIC CELLS

Dendritic cells are bone marrow-derived cells specialized for presenting antigens to either CD4[+] or CD8[+] T cells in order to initiate a primary immune response.

These cells appear to be generated from CD34[+] cells and require GM-CSF, TNFα, and possibly TGFβ for full maturation. Dendritic cells are found in all lymphoid tissues where they have specific names (Table 2-1). Because of their

TABLE 2-1
DENDRITIC AND OTHER PROFESSIONAL
ANTIGEN-PRESENTING CELLS

	LANGERHANS DENDRITIC CELL	INTER-DIGITATING CELL	FOLLICULAR DENDRITIC CELL	B CELL	MACRO-PHAGE
Location	Skin	Deep cortex, LN; PALS of spleen	Light zone of germinal centers	Cortex of LN; WP of spleen; 1° follicles	Mono-nuclear phagocytic system
Circulate in blood	−	−	−	+	+
$F_c \gamma R$	+	−	+	+	+
MHC class II	+	+	−	+	+
Phagocytic	−	−	−	±	+

highly efficient function in antigen presentation, they have come to be called "nature's adjuvant."

THYMUS

The thymus is a primary lymphoid organ that is required for the generation of immunocompetent $CD3^+4^+$ and $CD3^+8^+$ cells necessary for an adaptive immune response (Appendix 1).

The stroma of the thymus is composed of epithelial cells that originate from the third pharyngeal pouch in the embryo. The parenchyma is made up of thymocytes that are either positively and then negatively selected for maturation (<1%) or deleted (>99%) by apoptosis (Chap. 5). Most of the deletion of cells occurs in the cortex, with the medulla containing mainly mature cells.

After sIg^+ B cells, pre-T cells, monocytes, NK cells, and dendritic cells have developed in the marrow and $CD3^+4^+$ and $CD3^+8^+$ cells have matured in the thymus, they leave these primary lymphoid organs and migrate into peripheral secondary lymphoid tissue: lymph nodes spleen and mucosal associated lymphoid tissue.

LYMPH NODES

Lymph nodes (LNs) are encapsulated structures that are strategically placed throughout the body to receive and filter antigens and cells from peripheral interstitial fluid and lymph. All LNs eventually drain into the thoracic duct system and back to the peripheral blood.

There are approximately 550 kidney-shaped, 1–10 mm in diameter, lymph nodes in the body. Their indented hilus contains blood and lymphatic vessels (Fig. 2-2). Thus, LNs have two circulations, lymph and blood, which permeate a stroma of largely type III and I collagen. The type III collagen is arranged in a chicken wire fashion, forming lymphatic sinuses supporting a parenchyma of immunocompetent T and B cells as well as macrophages and other antigen-presenting cells. These cells are localized into:

1. **SUPERFICIAL CORTEX:** containing primary and secondary follicles with germinal centers containing dark and light zones (Fig. 11-1);
2. **DEEP CORTEX:** containing high endothelial post-capillary venules;
3. **MEDULLA:** with medullary cords.

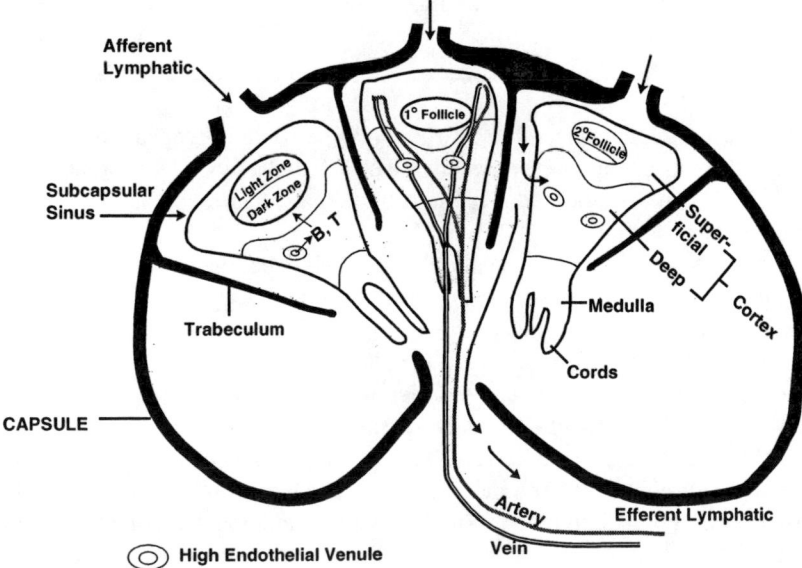

Figure 2-2
Structure of a lymph node.

Lymph enters a LN at its surface as numerous afferent lymphatics pierce its type I collagenous capsule and empty into the subcapsular sinus. It then percolates through the cortex into the medullary sinuses, where it leaves the hilus via efferent lymphatics. Any cells that enter through afferent lymphatics can also enter the parenchyma of the LN.

The hilar artery supplies the medulla and deep cortex but then empties into a capillary net on either side of the superficial cortical follicles. These capillaries then drain into post capillary venules (PCVs) with a very high cuboidal endothelium in the deep cortex. They then decrease their endothelial height, pass through the medulla, and leave the LN as hilar veins. It is at the PCVs in the deep cortex where circulating T and B cells adhere to PCV endothelium and migrate between these cells (diapedesis) into the node. Most B cells migrate superficially into follicles, with most of the T cells remaining in the deep cortex. They can remain in the LN for an undetermined period or enter a lymph sinus and exit via an efferent lymphatic. We will develop further the structure of the LN during an immune response in Chap. 11.

SPLEEN

The spleen is an encapsulated organ with lymphoid tissue called *white pulp* (*WP*), which can respond to blood-borne antigens surrounded by *red pulp* (*RP*). More lymphocytes circulate through it each day than any other secondary lymphoid organ.

Similar to LN, the spleen has a stroma of type III and I (capsule and trabecular) collagen that supports the parenchyma of WP and a blood sinusoidal system with cords of hemopoietic and lymphoid tissue called RP separated from each other by a marginal zone. (Fig. 2-3).

The part of the WP around a central arteriole is called the *periarteriolar lymphoid sheath* (*PALS*) and contains primarily T cells. It is thus analogous to the deep cortex of LN. The periphery of WP contains B cell-rich lymphoid follicles just like the periphery of LN. Between the periphery of the WP and the marginal zone is a blood filled marginal sinus, which receives capillary branches from the central arteriole. T and B cells leave the splenic circulation here and then migrate to the PALS or follicles, respectively. The marginal zone contains macrophages and some memory B cells. The marginal zone and sinus function as a part of B and T cell entry points into the WP similar to high endothelial venules of LN, but the marginal sinus has a low endothelium. B and T cells can migrate out of the WP into an RP cord through bridging channels (BCs) in the marginal zone.

The RP contains blood sinusoids with associated macrophages that line cellular cords. Some RP cords contain granulocytes, but others connect with WP fol-

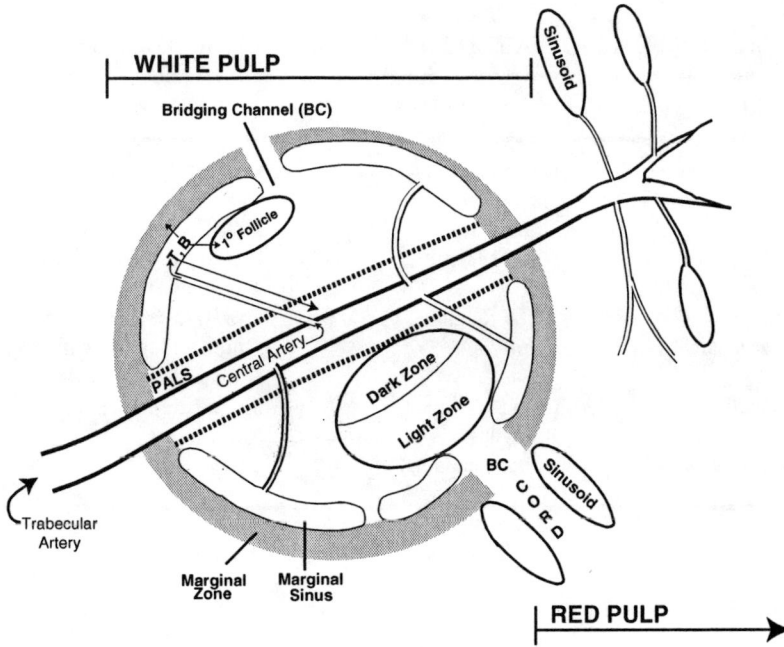

Figure 2-3
Structure of spleen white pulp with periarteriolar lymphoid sheath (PALS).

licles and contain plasma cells. The sinusoidal macrophages destroy old platelets and erythrocytes. The central arterioles empty directly into the RP cord or sinuses and then into trabecular veins.

MUCOSAL ASSOCIATED LYMPHOID TISSUE (MALT)

The epithelial lining, lamina propria, and submucosa of the gastrointestinal, respiratory, and genitourinary tracts contain wandering cells, diffuse aggregates, solitary primary nodules, or aggregates of secondary nodules that can become encapsulated. All of these are collectively called *mucosal associated lymphoid tissue (MALT)* (Table 2-2; Fig. 11-2).

While most of the diffuse and aggregated lymphoid tissue of the MALT is responsible for producing IgA, most intraepithelial lymphocytes (IEL) are CD8$^+$ $\alpha\beta$ (60%) or $\gamma\delta$ (40%) T cells. It appears that the $\gamma\delta$ cells may react to bacterial hsp65. The epithelial lining over Peyer's patches (PP) contains specialized antigen-transporting cells called *M cells*, which transport luminal antigen to under-

TABLE 2-2
MUCOSAL ASSOCIATED LYMPHOID TISSUE (MALT)

ORGAN	LOCATION	EPITHELIUM
GALT	Gastrointestinal tract	
Tonsils		
Palatine	Oral pharynx	Stratified squamous
Pharyngeal	Nasopharynx	Pseudostratified ciliated columnar
Lingual	Distal tongue	Stratified squamous
Peyer's patches	Ileum	Simple columnar with microfold (M) cells
Appendix	Colon	Simple columnar
BALT-LUNG	Bronchus	Respiratory
GENITOURINARY	Ureter, bladder	Transitional

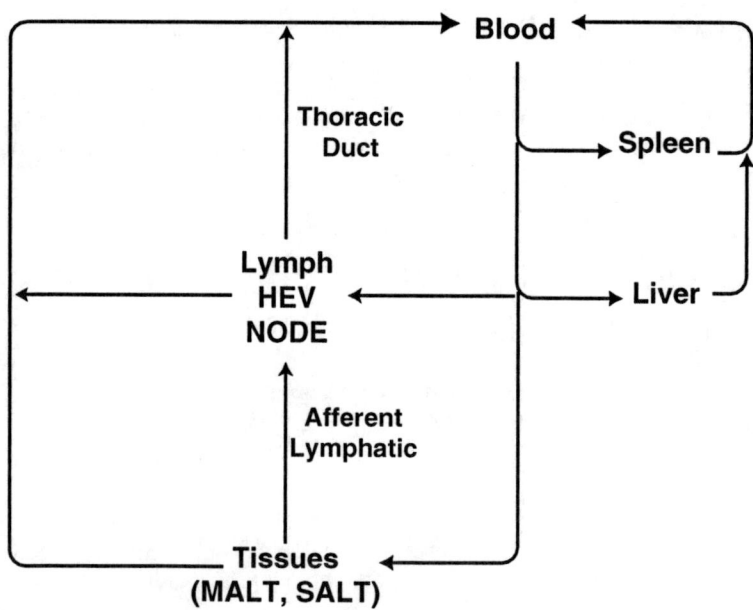

Figure 2-4
Lymphocyte recirculation.

lying antigen reactive lymphocytes. It should also be realized that most of the cells activated in the MALT stay in or return to the MALT. Thus, cells stimulated in PP or tonsils enter mesenteric or cervical lymph nodes for further maturation. After re-entering the circulation, they home back to the MALT.

CIRCULATION AND RECIRCULATION

Both T and B cells continuously circulate and recirculate, blood → lymph → blood. Approximately 1–2% recirculate every hour (Fig. 2-4). However, NK cells are only found in blood, spleen, and liver.

ANTIGEN AND ANTIBODY STRUCTURE
PART A: ANTIGEN

•

- **Antigen**
- **Immunogen**
- **Hapten**
- **Factors That Determine the Immunogenic Potential of an Antigen**

• • • • • • • • • • • • •

ANTIGEN

An antigen is a molecule that binds to a specific protein structure called an *antibody*.

An antigen binds to a specific antibody to provide a mechanism by which the antigen is recognized and inactivated. In this manner, an antigen complexes with a specific antibody so that the complex can attach itself to specialized immune cells that either internalize the complex to destroy it or release biologic mediators such as histamine to induce an allergic/inflammatory response.

The binding process of antigen to specific antibody forms the basis of a test called an enzyme-linked immunosorbent assay (ELISA) that can be used to measure the amount of antigen in a biological fluid. As shown in Fig. 3-1, a sample of biological fluid such as blood serum is placed into a solid support vesicle that has been coated with an antibody that specifically recognizes a specific part of some antigen found in blood. This antigen binds to the coating antibody and is detected by the addition of another antibody that specifically recognizes another specific part of the antigen that is bound to the coating antibody. This detecting antibody is linked to an enzyme that specifically reacts with a substrate that is

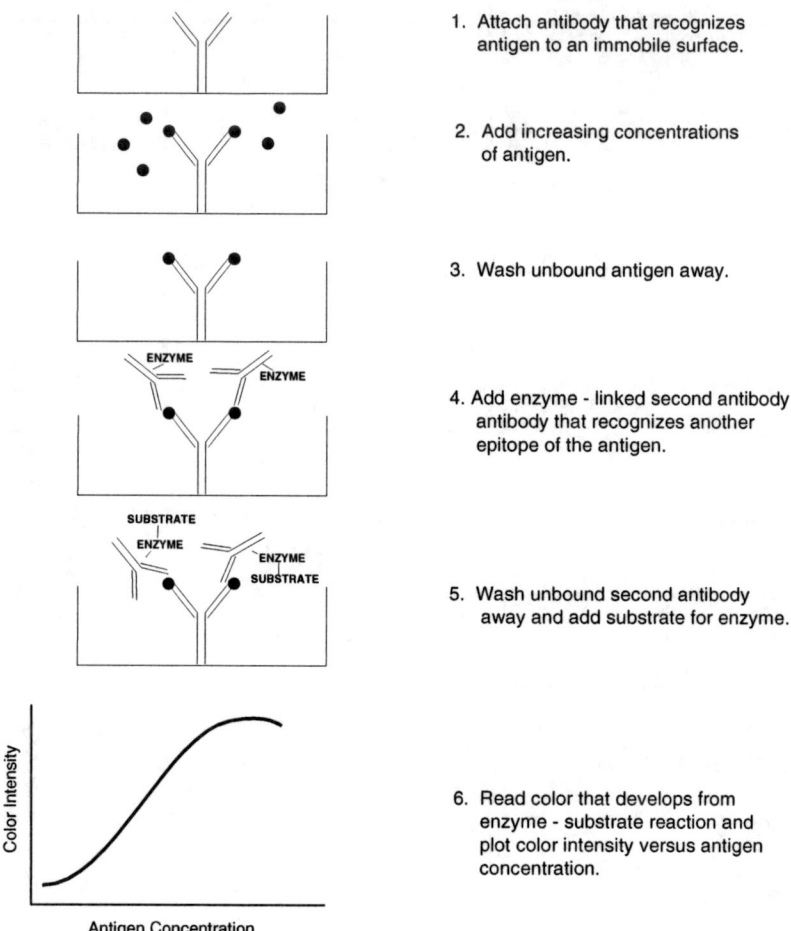

Figure 3-1
Schematic of the enzyme-linked immunosorbent assay (ELISA).

then added to the reaction mixture to yield a colored solution. The color intensity of the solution is indicative of the amount of antigen in the fluid sample (i.e., the darker the color, the greater the amount of antigen present in the assayed sample). Thus, the binding of an antigen to a specific antibody provides the physician with a means to measure the concentration of a specific antigen in biological fluids.

IMMUNOGEN

An immunogen is an antigen that activates immune cells to generate an immune response against itself. Thus, an immunogen is an antigen, but an antigen is not necessarily an immunogen.

By itself, penicillin is an antigen that can bind to a specific antibody, but it is not immunogenic; i.e., it cannot activate immune cells to elicit an immune response to produce those specific antibodies. In order to be immunogenic, penicillin must first become a chemically reactive molecule, such as penicilloic acid, that is able to covalently attach itself to an endogenous carrier protein, such as serum albumin or other cell surface membrane proteins (Fig. 3-2). In this manner, the penicilloic acid-protein molecule becomes an immunogen that is capable of activating both T and B lymphocytes to elicit the production of antibodies by B cells that are able to specifically bind to penicillin, the antigen. It should be pointed out that the terms *antigen* and *immunogen* are often used interchangeably in most textbooks and journal articles, but an understanding of the conceptual difference between the two terms is critical to understanding the mechanism by which immune responses are generated against antigens.

HAPTEN

A hapten is a small organic molecule that is not immunogenic by itself.

In order to study the specificity of antigen binding by antibody molecules, researchers have synthesized small organic molecules whose structures can be specifically modified at specific sites. For example, benzene rings with either nitroso or arsonate groups at different positions in the ring possess only one site for the binding of an antibody and are referred to as *haptens*. Using a specific hapten coupled to an immunogenic protein carrier, a specific antibody can be produced that either binds strongly to that specific hapten alone, and not to related haptens, or binds strongly to that specific hapten, and weakly to related haptens (Fig. 3-3). The latter finding provides a mechanistic basis for the ability of an antibody to bind other molecules that closely resemble a particular antigenic structure (i.e., a cross-reacting antibody). Other examples of haptens include nucleic acids, phospholipids, and small molecular weight molecules such as penicillin.

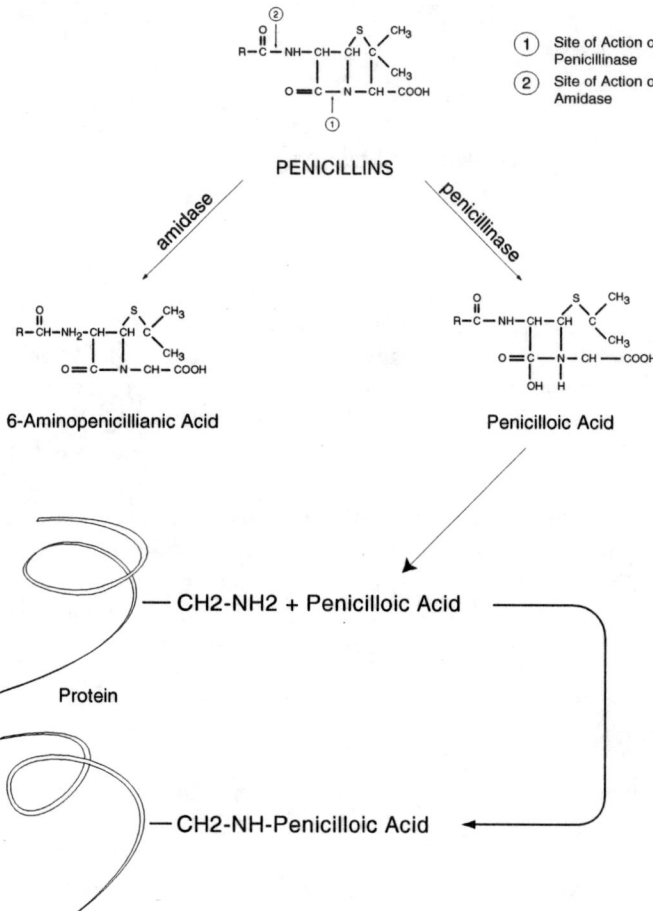

Figure 3-2
Penicilloic acid-protein conjugate
Penicilloic acid groups can be readily conjugated to proteins. Conjugation usually takes place to the amino groups of lysine.

Outside of the laboratory, haptens pose a serious health risk to humans. This risk has increased dramatically in recent years, since humans are exposed to an ever increasing number of haptens in their environment. When these haptens gain entry into the host, they may complex with host proteins to create immunogenic hapten-protein molecules. In this manner, an environmental hapten, such as nickel, may initially complex with host proteins and elicit the initial production

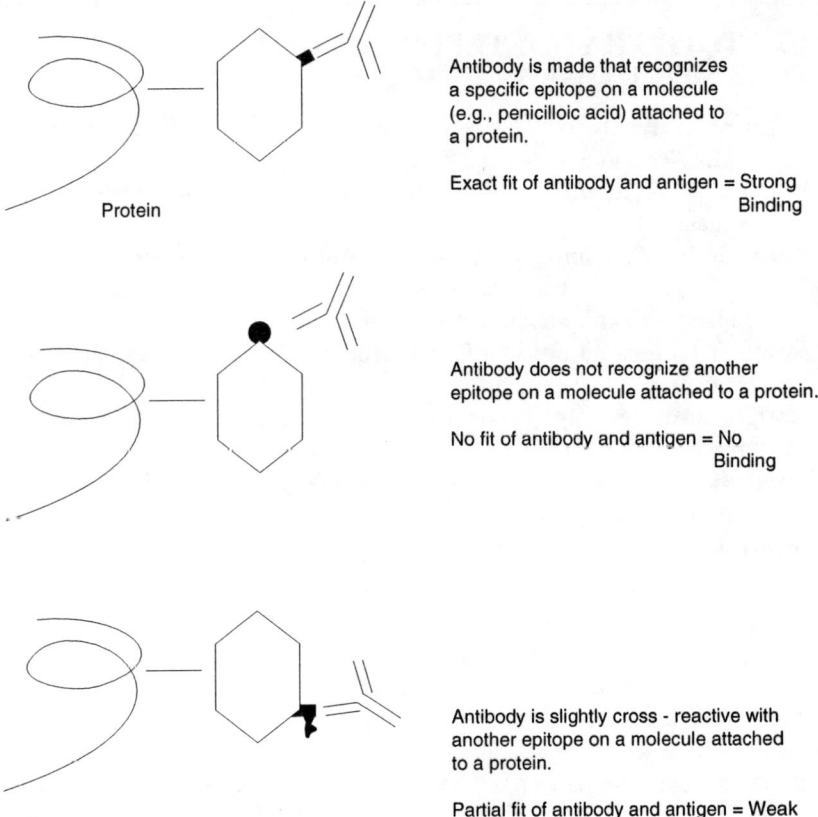

Antibody is made that recognizes
a specific epitope on a molecule
(e.g., penicilloic acid) attached to
a protein.

Exact fit of antibody and antigen = Strong
Binding

Protein

Antibody does not recognize another
epitope on a molecule attached to a protein.

No fit of antibody and antigen = No
Binding

Antibody is slightly cross - reactive with
another epitope on a molecule attached
to a protein.

Partial fit of antibody and antigen = Weak
Binding

Figure 3-3
Binding affinity of antibody.

of antibodies against the hapten. However, upon reexposure to nickel, two separate reactions can occur. One reaction is protective and involves the production
of antibodies that bind to the hapten and clear it from the circulation. The other
reaction is pathological and involves the binding of antigen to specific IgE antibody (see Chap. 12) that is attached to mast cells, precipitating histamine release
and an allergic response. Thus, haptens are small nonimmunogenic antigens that
can be made into immunogens that can elicit either clinical or pathological
immune reactions.

FACTORS THAT DETERMINE THE IMMUNOGENIC POTENTIAL OF AN ANTIGEN

Degree of foreignness: degree to which a molecule is different from molecules normally found in the body.

Distance in phylogenetic relationship: mouse cells are immunogenic in humans.

Accessibility of an antigenic epitope to immune cell recognition: epitopes on the outside of a structure are strongly immunogenic; epitopes within a structure are weakly immunogenic.

Route of antigen administration: IV for particulate antigens; subcutaneous for soluble antigens.

Antigen dose: very high or low doses may induce a state of nonresponsiveness.

Frequency of antigen administration: multiple administrations of antigen make the antigen more immunogenic.

Adjuvants: augment the immunogenicity of a soluble antigen.

The immunogenic potential of an antigen can be determined by either the *degree of foreignness* of the antigenic molecule to the host or the *distance in phylogenetic relationship* between the antigenic molecule and the host. For example, the molecules that make up both a host cell surface and biological fluid are considered a part of *self* and, therefore, are not immunogenic. However, *non-self* molecules are characterized as 1) molecules, such as penicillin, that can become chemically reactive and attach to proteins; 2) molecules expressed on the surface of a transformed cancer cell in the host; 3) molecules expressed by protein molecules from another species, such as serum albumin (for example, although albumin is a critical component of blood serum and the amino acid sequence of albumin from two species is similar, a few minor amino acid differences do exist. It is these minor amino acid differences that make rabbit albumin foreign and, therefore, immunogenic to humans); or 4) molecules normally associated with only the interior of a host cell and not normally exposed on the cell surface. For example, myelin basic proteins are a major component of Schwann cells and oligodendrocytes, but they are not normally expressed on the cell surface. However, after nerve injury, myelin basic proteins are exposed and are now recognized as non-self because they had never been seen by the immune system before. Thus, *non-self* is a misleading term, since myelin basic proteins are indeed a part of *self*. But, nonetheless, it is a term that is often used to describe immunogens vs. nonimmunogens.

It is important to note that a single antigen may be capable of binding different specific antibodies. This is because the antigen may contain one or more different antigenic determinants, called *epitopes*, each of which is capable of binding to a specific antibody. For example, a complex microorganism, such as a virus, contains many different epitopes, some of which will be strongly immunogenic, while others will be weakly immunogenic. The degree of immunogenicity of each epitope depends on the *accessibility of each epitope to recognition* by cells of the immune system that will generate an immune response against the specific epitope. Hydrophilic groups on molecules, such as the ends of amino acid chains or carbohydrate side chains, are strong immunogenic epitopes, while hydrophobic groups, such as molecules hidden within a complex molecular structure, are weak immunogenic epitopes. Such weakly immunogenic antigens must be partially degraded so that the hidden immunogenic determinants can be exposed (to be discussed in more detail in Chap. 7).

Other factors that determine the degree of immunogenicity of a given antigen include the *route of antigen administration, antigen dose*, frequency of antigen administration, and use of adjuvant. For example, particulate antigens, such as bacteria and viruses, are more immunogenic when they are administered intravenously. In contrast, soluble antigens, such as proteins, nucleic acids, and carbohydrates, are more immunogenic when administered subcutaneously. Also, antigens given orally (parenterally) may elicit immune responses in the gut that allow for the production of antibodies that protect us from the antigen crossing the gut lining and entering the internal compartments of the body. However, parenterally administered antigens may also induce a state of tolerance to the antigen if it should gain entry to the internal environment a second time via another route in an appropriate dose. This latter phenomenon may be related to the finding that very low or very high doses of antigen are not able to elicit a strong immune response and may actually induce a state of immune nonresponsiveness/tolerance in the host. This nonresponsive/tolerogenic state of immune cells will be discussed in more detail in Chap. 16. In contrast, intermediate doses of antigen elicit strong immune responses that provide protection to the host against the antigen.

The *frequency of antigen administration* also determines the magnitude of the immune response that is generated against an antigen. Most antigens require several administrations to achieve optimal immunogenicity. For example, a primary administration of antigen elicits a primary immune response of a given magnitude. A second administration of the antigen elicits a secondary response that is of a higher magnitude as compared with the primary response. A third administration of the antigen elicits an even greater immune response. The mechanisms by which these immune responses increase in magnitude will be discussed in Chap. 9.

And finally, the immunogenicity of soluble antigens can be augmented when they are administered in conjunction with compounds known as *adjuvants*. Adjuvants, such as killed mycobacteria or *Bordetella pertussis*, help to augment the immune response that is generated against a particular antigen. The mechanisms responsible for the action of adjuvants are not well understood at present, but they probably involve the activation of antigen-presenting cells, such as macrophages, for efficient antigen uptake and processing for the presentation of degraded immunogenic peptides to T cells.

In the subsequent section of this chapter and in other chapters, we will learn about the production by B lymphocytes of antibodies that are directed against an antigen as well as the mechanisms by which specific antibody isotypes and affinities are produced and the clinical significance of their production.

PART B: ANTIBODY

•

- **Antibodies or Immunoglobulins**
- **Isotypes**
- **Hypervariable Region**
- **Allotypes**
- **Idiotypes**
- **Papain**
- **Pepsin**

• • • • • • • • • • • • •

ANTIBODIES OR IMMUNOGLOBULINS

Antibodies or immunoglobulins (Ig) are glycoproteins produced by plasma cells and are present in the γ globulin fraction of serum. Each Ig is composed of two 200-amino acid-long identical light (L) chains (each with a molecular mass of 24 kD) linked via disulfide bonds to two 400-amino acid-long polypeptide heavy (H) chains (each ranging from 55 to 70 kD). There are five classes or *isotypes* of Ig, which differ because of five potential variations in the amino acid sequences in the carboxy-terminal portion of their H chains, thus producing IgM, IgG, IgE, IgA, and IgD isotypes (Table 3-1). IgG has four subclasses (IgG1–4) based on some further structural differences in their γ1–4 type of H chains. IgA has two subclasses, IgA1 and IgA2, which are designated as 1 and 2 based on their serum concentration.

TABLE 3-1
Ig CLASS AND SUBCLASS DEPEND ON H CHAIN TYPE

Ig CLASS	Ig SUBCLASS	H CHAIN TYPE	ALLOTYPE
IgM	—	μ	—
IgD	—	δ	—
IgG		γ	—
	IgG1	$\gamma 1$	G1m 1–4, 17
	IgG2	$\gamma 2$	G2m 23
	IgG3	$\gamma 3$	G3m 5, 6, 11, 13–16, 21
	IgG4	$\gamma 4$	G4m,
IgE	—	ϵ	—
IgA		α	—
	IgA1	$\alpha 1$	—
	IgA2	$\alpha 2$	A2m 1, 2

ISOTYPES

There are two isotypes of L chains (κ or λ) based on structural differences, with each Ig molecule containing either two κ or two λ but never a mixture. The L chain has two domains: one C_L at the C-terminal part and one V_L at the N-terminal end, which is part of the antigen-binding site (Figs. 3-4 and 3-5).

The five isotypes of H chains (μ, γ, ϵ, α, δ) each contain three or four C_H domains at the C-terminal end and one V_H at the N-terminal end (Table 3-2). There may be a hinge region between the CH_1 and CH_2 regions. The C region also contains sites for binding complement (C′), the F_c receptors on monocytes, macrophages, B cells, and mast cells as well as the sites that bind to and cross the placenta (Fig. 3-5).

There can be from 1 to 15 interchain (H-L, H-H, L-L) disulfide (-S-S) bonds depending on the isotype or subclass of Ig molecule, but only one S-S bond connects H and L chains. L chains have two intrachain -S-S bonds. However, γ, α, and δ H chains have four and μ and ϵ have five.

HYPERVARIABLE REGION

Both H and L chains have a V region, but there are particular areas in this region where the amino acid sequences are highly variable. These *hypervariable* areas in the V regions are called complementary determining regions (CDRs) because they are important in determining the structure of the antigen-binding site (paratope).

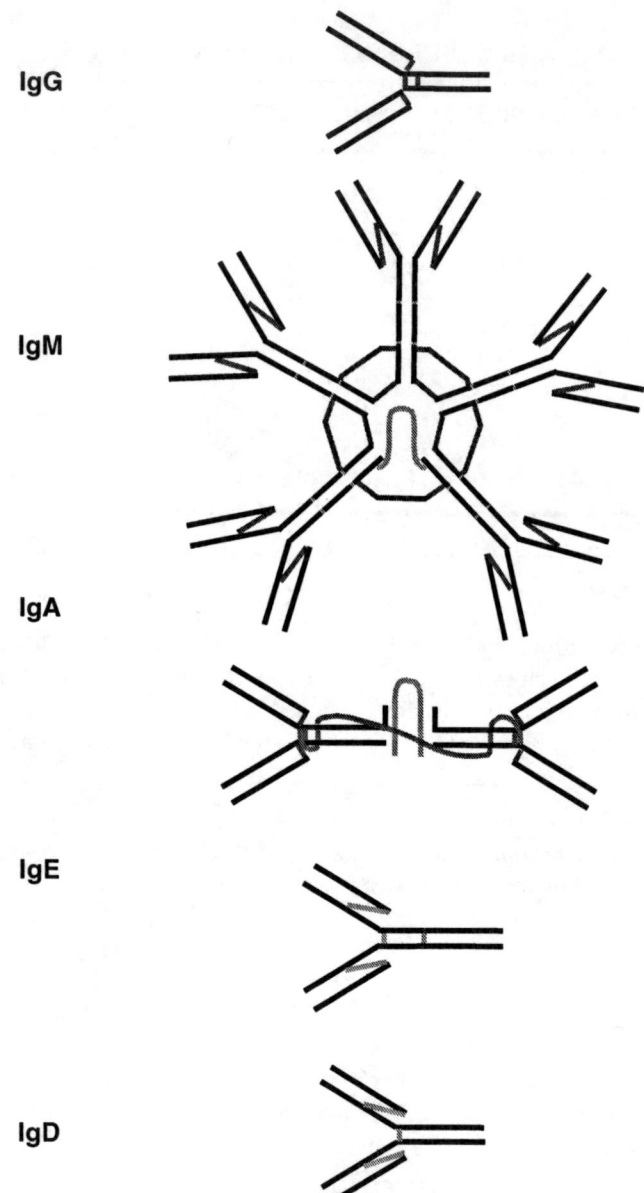

IgG

IgM

IgA

IgE

IgD

Figure 3-4
Ig isotype structure.

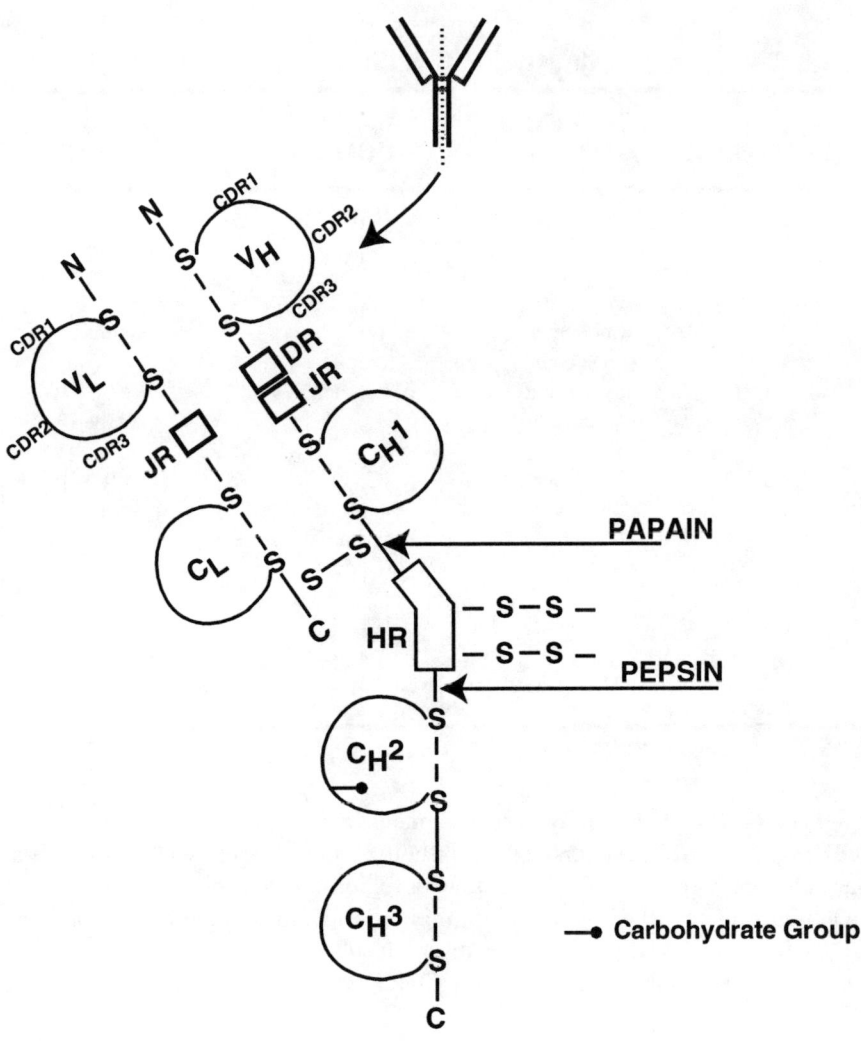

Figure 3-5
Schematic of Ig molecule with papain and pepsin proteolytic sites.

TABLE 3-2
MAJOR FIVE Ig ISOTYPES

ISOTYPE	SECRETED FORM	H CHAIN DOMAINS	MASS
IgG	Monomer	$3C_H$, $1V_H$	$\sim 1.5 \times 10^5$ daltons
IgM	Pentamer (monomer on B cells)	$4C_H$, $1V_H$ ↑ Carbo-hydrate	$\sim 9 \times 10^5$ daltons
IgA	Dimer and J chain	$3C_H$, and $1V_H$	$\sim 1.6 \times 10^5$ daltons
IgE	Monomer	$4C_H$, $1V_H$ ↑ Carbo-hydrate	$\sim 1.9 \times 10^5$ daltons
IgD	Monomer	$3C_H$, $1V_H$	$\sim 1.8 \times 10^5$ daltons

The *CDRs* are short polypeptide segments close to amino acid positions 30 (CDR1), 50 (CDR2), and 95 (CDR3) for both H and L chains. CDR3 is the most variable. Between the CDRs are framework regions, which are relatively constant in amino acid sequence. When the V region is folded in three dimensions, the CDRs loop out toward the apex of the molecule but lie in close proximity to form the antigen-binding surface with CDR1 lying between CDR3 and CDR2 (Fig. 3-5).

ALLOTYPES

While there are five Ig H chain isotypes within the same individual, allelic variants by a few amino acids exist between individuals of the same species, which are inherited in a Mendelian manner. The different forms of a gene for a particular locus determining the amino acid composition of Ig H and L chains in each individual are called *allotypes* (Table 3-1).

C'FIX	SERUM CONCENTRATION	FUNCTION
Variable	~1200 mg/dl	Produced in 2° response to T-dependent (TD) Ag; crosses placenta
Effective (classical pathway)	~100 mg/dl	Produced in 1° response to TDAg; 1° in response to T-independent Ag
Effective (alternate pathway)	~300 mg/dl	Mucosal immunity
—	~30μg/dl	Allergic hypersensitivity: attach to $F_c\epsilon$ receptor on mast cells and basophils
—	~3 mg/dl	B cell Ag receptor along with monomeric IgM

There are allotype-specific antibodies, which can detect these differences in H and L chains between individuals. H chain allotypic markers are designated gamma markers (Gm) and alpha markers (Am) for the γH and αH chains. γH has four different isotypes, γ1–4, and each has a series of distinct allotypic markers designated G1m (1, 2, 3, 4, 17), G2m23, G3m (5, 6, 11, 13, 14, 15, 16, 21), and G4m (4a, 4b). αH has only two alleles at its locus, designated A1m and A2m. There are three alleles at the κL locus, designated Km1, Km2, Km3. These three vary only in single amino acids at positions 153 and 191 from the N-terminal end. Allotypic markers have been used to help resolve some medicolegal issues such as paternity typing and blood stain origins. They also can help verify B cell engraftment after bone marrow transplantation.

IDIOTYPES

Idiotypes are unique antigenic determinants (epitopes) present in or close to the antigen combining site of H and L chains. Thus, the hypervariable CDR1–3 regions that actually make contact with the epitope of the antigen may themselves act as antigenic determinants (idiotopes), and the idiotype of an Ig is the idiotope.

Thus, it is possible to induce the production of anti-idiotypic (a-ID) antibodies that structurally resemble the original epitope in that they actually resemble an internal image of the epitope. These a-ID antibodies could be used to induce production of the original antibodies in an unimmunized recipient.

PAPAIN

Papain is a proteolytic enzyme that splits IgG molecules into three fragments just proximal to the hinge region. Two identical fragments contain an intact L chain attached to the V_H-$C\gamma1$ part of the H chain. Because they can still bind Ag, they are called Fab (fragment Ag-binding). The third piece contains identical fragments of the $C\gamma2$ and $C\gamma3$ domains joined at the hinge region. This piece can readily crystallize and is called the F_c (fragment crystallizable). The F_c piece of the antibody is what binds to F_c receptors on certain cells and activates complement (Fig. 3-2).

PEPSIN

Pepsin is also a proteolytic enzyme that cleaves IgG molecules at the carboxyl terminus of the hinge region near the $C\gamma2$ domain. Thus, the hinge region and interchain disulfide bonds are retained in an $F(ab')_2$ molecule, but the F_c fragment is degraded.

B CELL DEVELOPMENT

·

- **B Cells Develop in the Bone Marrow**
- **Rearrangement of Immunoglobulin Genes**
- **Recombination Enzymes RAG-1 and RAG-2**
- **The Pre-B Cell Receptor: An Ig Expressed by Early B Cells**
- **Selection of Immature B Cells**
- **Immunoglobulin Genes Are Fully Rearranged Only in B Cells**
- **Sources of Antibody Diversity**

· · · · · · · · · · · · · ·

B CELLS DEVELOP IN THE BONE MARROW

B lymphocytes are formed in the hematopoietic tissues of mammals, first in the *fetal liver* and finally the *bone marrow*. B cells originate from the multipotent hematopoietic stem cells that give rise to all blood cell types.

B lymphopoiesis is generally defined as the generation of a pool of mature B cells with a large diversity of receptors for many different antigens. Each B cell's antigen receptor (immunoglobulin, Ig) must display monospecificity, so that each B cell can produce antibody of only one specificity. Cells that are committed to the B cell lineage in the bone marrow express cell surface glycoproteins CD45RA (B220) and CD19 (Appendix 1).

Two events hallmark the formation of B lymphocytes in the marrow before their exit to peripheral lymphoid tissues: *sequential somatic gene rearrangement* of the heavy and light chain genes for immunoglobulin and *expression of a characteristic pattern of cell surface and intracellular molecules* that regulate differentiation.

The expression of cell surface molecules has allowed the recognition of distinct stages of B cell differentiation. However, it should be realized that the

TABLE 4-1
STAGES IN THE DEVELOPMENT OF A B LYMPHOCYTE

STAGE	CHROMOSOMAL Ig GENE REARRANGEMENTS		Ig PROTEIN EXPRESSED
	IgH	IgL	
Pre-pro	DJ/GL	GL/GL	None
Early pro	DJ/DJ	GL/GL	None
Late pro	VDJ/DJ	GL/GL	Pre-B cell receptor
Pre	VDJ/DJ	VJ/GL	Igμ
Newly formed	VDJ/DJ	VJ/GL	IgM
Mature	VDJ/DJ	VJ/GL	IgM, IgD

GL: germline.

process is a continuous one so that division into stages is somewhat arbitrary (Table 4-1).

B lymphopoiesis occurs throughout the lifetime of humans and rodents. Proliferation of the precursor stages is a key element in regulation of B cell production. Nonhematopoietic fibroblastic-like cells, called *stromal cells*, make up the microenvironment that controls commitment of stem cells into the B cell lineage and numbers of lymphocytes produced per day. Stromal cells form a reticular network of cell processes that contact millions of hematopoietic precursors of all lineages. At early stages, the B cell precursors (pre-pro-B cells) must interact physically with the stromal cells in order for proliferation and maturation to occur. Later stages (late pro-B cells) merely need the soluble growth factors produced by stromal cells. Stromal cells produce several necessary growth factors and cell-cell adhesion molecules. One key growth factor for B lymphopoiesis is *interleukin-7*. Mice that lack either interleukin-7 or its receptor are vastly deficient in B cells and serum antibodies.

REARRANGEMENT OF IMMUNOGLOBULIN GENES

The process of *immunoglobulin gene rearrangement* has been studied extensively. Ig rearrangement is a highly ordered process that is similar to T cells (Chap. 5) but ensures that only B lymphocytes will produce immunoglobulin.

The earliest identifiable stage of B cell differentiation is the *pre-pro-B cell*. In this stage, the process of Ig gene rearrangement begins. The first rearrangement entails the joining of the D segment to the J segment of the *Ig heavy chain gene (IgH)*. Subsequent rearrangements bring the V region juxtaposed to the DJ portion (see Fig. 4-2). A productive rearrangement of the IgH gene must occur before rearrangement of the *Ig light chain gene (IgL)* will begin.

The *pro-B cell* stage is highlighted by continued IgH rearrangement, joining the V region with the already joined DJ segments. While the DJ rearrangements take place on both chromosomes, VDJ rearrangement usually occurs only on one chromosome. If the rearrangement is not productive, for example due to introduction of a new stop codon or frame shift, rearrangement then proceeds to the second chromosome. By the end of the pro-B stage, IgH rearrangement is complete.

By the time the cells reach the *pre-B cell* stage, Igμ protein can be observed in the cytoplasm, and rearrangement of one of the two *immunoglobulin light chain (IgL)* genes initiates. The method of rearrangement is similar, but only one joining is needed to bring the V region sequence to the J segment. The rearrangement begins first on the kappa gene, and if this is unproductive, then the lambda genes are rearranged.

RECOMBINATION ENZYMES RAG-1 AND RAG-2

Two proteins necessary for the rearrangement process, *RAG-1* and *RAG-2* (recombinase-activating genes 1 and 2), appear at the pre-pro-B cell stage. RAG-1 and RAG-2 genes are active during all phases of Ig gene rearrangement, but these genes are not expressed in mature B cells that have completed rearrangement. However, Ag-activated B cells in the germinal center reexpress *RAG* genes as the cells undergo affinity maturation (Chap. 11).

Terminal deoxynucleotidal transferase (TdT) is another enzyme that is involved in IgH rearrangement and is expressed early in the formation of B cells, but it is not necessary for rearrangement to take place. When TdT is present, random nucleotides are added to open N regions during the rearrangement of D and J segments, thus increasing the diversity of the sequences. The expression of TdT diminishes by the late pro-B cell stage, prior to light chain rearrangement. TdT is a marker of leukemic cells of early B and T lineage origin. TdT is expressed by normal B cell precursors only during the stage of IgH gene rearrangement. Consequently, IgH but not IgL shows N region diversity.

THE PRE-B CELL RECEPTOR: AN Ig EXPRESSED BY EARLY B CELLS

Two transiently expressed proteins were discovered recently that form a light chain-like molecule termed the *surrogate light chain*. The surrogate light chain is composed of two gene products, lambda 5 and V-pre-B, which respectively are homologous with the lambda IgL and V region genes. Surrogate light chains can combine with the μ heavy chain protein in pro- and pre-B cells, forming a structure referred to as the *pre-B cell receptor*. The combination of the IgH protein and the surrogate light chains may be involved in stimulating proliferation of cells in the late pro-B cell stage of differentiation. Few B cells form in the absence of the pre-B cell receptor. After kappa or lambda light chain proteins are synthesized, the IgL displaces the surrogate light chain from interaction with the IgH protein so that the intact immunoglobulin can be formed and delivered to the cell surface.

SELECTION OF IMMATURE B CELLS

A *newly formed B cell* displays IgM on the cell surface. At this stage, the B cell is still immature and responds to antigen differently from a mature B cell. Immature B cells can be functionally removed by interaction with self antigen, either by undergoing *programmed cell death* (apoptosis) or by *anergy*, in which the cell is rendered nonresponsive in the presence of the antigen. Thus, similar to T cells (Chap. 5), immature B lymphocytes undergo a process of "negative selection" to delete cells that are reactive to "self" antigens.

Immature B cells that are not removed by the processes of negative selection leave the bone marrow and migrate to peripheral or secondary lymphoid tissues such as the spleen and lymph nodes. Here further maturation takes place and the newly formed B cells express IgD, in addition to IgM, on the cell surface. The mature B cells are now fully responsive to antigens and interaction with T cells. When they interact with antigen in secondary lymphoid tissue, they, as well as some Th cells, help form germinal centers, whereupon somatic hypermutation, selection of cells producing high affinity antibody, class switching, and production of plasmablasts as well as memory cells occurs (Chap. 11).

The tissue-specific regulation of Ig gene rearrangement occurs on several levels. First, the Ig gene chromatin "opens" and becomes accessible for transcription. The accessibility of the chromatin is necessary for recombination and is controlled by tissue-specific transcription factors. Second, recombination signal sequences, conserved monomer/heptamer sequences, flank the V, D, and J segments of the heavy chain gene and V and J segments of the light chain genes. The juxtaposition of these sequences brings the two recombining segments into close proximity and makes the intervening DNA into a loop that can be cleaved by recombination-specific enzymes. The limited tissue expression of two of the enzymes necessary for recombination, RAG-1 and RAG-2, is a third level of regulation. Thus, only in B cells are fully rearranged Ig heavy or light chain genes observed (Figs. 4-1 and 4-2).

IMMUNOGLOBULIN GENES ARE FULLY REARRANGED ONLY IN B CELLS

Tissue-specific transcription factors regulate accessibility of the Ig gene chromatin.

Ig gene segments are flanked by unique recombination signal sequences.

Expression of recombination enzymes is highly regulated in lymphoid cells.

The *monospecificity* of each newly formed B cell is achieved by the sum processes of cellular differentiation. This phenomenon is called *allelic exclusion*, referring to the fact only the Ig genes on one allele (chromosome) are transcribed and translated into protein. This assures that one B cell will react with only one antigenic determinant and will produce antibody to only that antigen.

The somatic recombination of Ig heavy and light chain gene segments accounts for the extreme *diversity of the B cell antigen repertoire*. In the heavy chain gene, any of four J region segments may combine with any of 15 D segments, and the VD product may combine with any of more than 200 V genes. Diversity is expanded by the imprecise joining of the DNA or even the addition

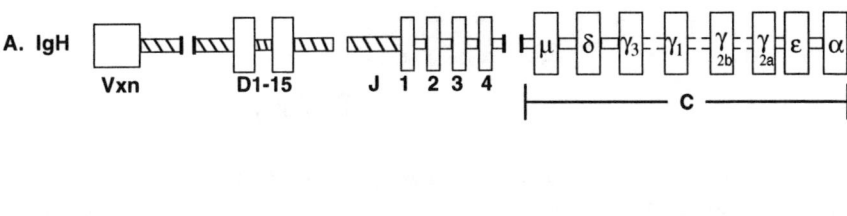

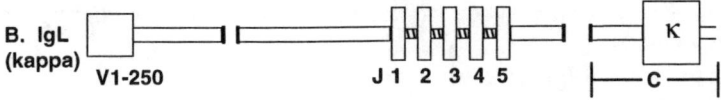

Figure 4-1
Organization of Ig genes.

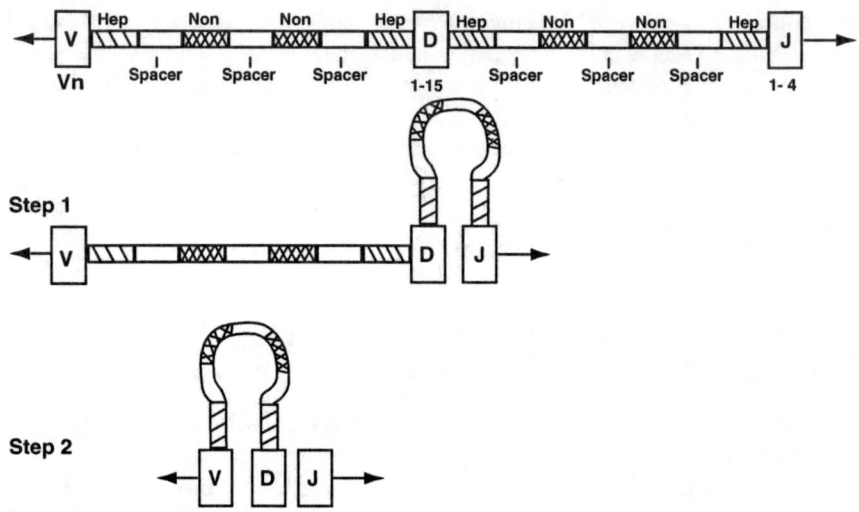

Figure 4-2
VDJ joining.

of random nucleotides by TdT during rearrangement. Even more diversity is added by the order of rearrangements. The heavy chain genes rearrange prior to the light chain genes. Once a productive heavy chain rearrangement is achieved, a phase of rapid cellular division occurs, which produces several daughter cells expressing identical Ig heavy chains. The daughter cells each produce different light chain gene rearrangements and, subsequently, proteins that combine with the heavy chain proteins to yield many unique antigen-binding specificities. In this manner, as many as 10^{11} different antibody specificities can be generated in the primary repertoire from newly formed B cells. However, it should be realized that further selection for high affinity antibody-producing cells will occur in the germinal centers of secondary lymphoid tissue.

SOURCES OF ANTIBODY DIVERSITY

Multiple D and J genes can combine into many different patterns with up to 200 V genes.

Rejoining of the DNA cleavage sites may yield codons for new amino acid sequences.

TdT adds nucleotides to the N regions of the DNA that are cleaved during recombination.

Combining of identical IgH proteins with different IgL chains yields multiple specificities.

THE THYMUS AND T CELL DEVELOPMENT

•

- **Thymic Tissue Architecture**
- **T Cell Developmental Stages in the Thymus**
- **Physical Structures of T Cell Receptor (TCR) Genes**
- **T Cell Selection in the Thymus**
- **Major Histocompatibility Complex (MHC) Restriction**
- **Transgenic Mice**

•   •   •   •   •   •   •   •   •   •   •   •

As we discussed in Chap. 4, the immune cells that synthesize and secrete Ig are termed B cells. The identification of B cells comes from the observation that removing the bursa (bursectomy) of Fabricius, a secondary lymphoid organ in birds, totally ablates the ability to produce antibody. In contrast, the ability to reject a foreign skin graft is intact in bursectomized birds. However, removing the thymus gland (thymectomy) in newborn mice subsequently prolongs skin graft survival and reduces an antibody response to specific antigens. From these results, it is clear that there are at least two types of immune cells: B cells, which produce Ig and participate in the antibody or humoral immune response, and T cells, which develop in the thymus and are responsible for skin graft rejection and other cell-mediated immune responses. Furthermore, a reduction in antibody responses in thymectomized animals indicates that B cells do not function independently but rather require the cooperation of T cells (T cell help). In this chapter we will learn about the tissue architecture of the thymus and the developmental stages of T cells within this organ.

THYMIC TISSUE ARCHITECTURE

The thymus is made up of various cell types derived from various origins. Histologically, the thymus has three distinct components: the *subcapsular cortex*, the *cortex*, and the *medulla*. Developing T cells or thymocytes are found embedded in an epithelial network known as the *thymic stroma*. Abnormal development of thymic stroma results in severe depletion of mature T cells and immunodeficiency diseases.

In both mice and humans, the thymus is a bilobed organ that is located just above the heart, anterior to all the great blood vessels, but its location in other vertebrates varies. For example, in birds, the thymus is located along the neck area. Histologically, this organ is compartmentalized into incomplete lobules; each is delineated by an outer layer of connective tissue, or capsule, and interlobular connective tissue, or septum. Within each lobule, one can clearly identify the outer dense **thymic cortex**, packed with T cells of the thymus, or *thymocytes*, and the inner *thymic medulla* with fewer thymocytes and *Hassall's corpuscles*, a specialized group of medullary epithelial cells. The epithelial cell layer that is proximal to the capsule and septum is known as the *subcapsular cortex*, and the area between the deep thymic cortex and the medulla is referred to as the *cortical-medullary junction*. The cortical-medullary junction is where precursor cells enter and migrate toward the subcapsular cortical region. T cells mature in the cortex and then migrate toward the medulla. Mature T cells then exit from the medulla to the peripheral circulation via postcapillary venules and lymphatics. The developing thymocytes within the cortex and the mature T cells in the medulla are embedded in an epithelial network known as the *thymic stroma* that makes up a unique thymic microenvironment necessary for T cell development (Table 5-1). The thymic epithelial cell network can be visualized by staining with antibodies that detect keratin, a group of cytoskeletal proteins specific for epithelial cells. During embryonic development, the thymic epithelium forms a rudimentary thymus, or *thymic anlage*, which attracts hematopoietic cells first from the yolk sac, then from fetal liver, and later from the bone marrow. The cells that colonize the thymic anlage include precursor T cells, dendritic cells or interdigitating cells, and macrophages (see Table 5-1).

Abnormal development of the thymic anlage results in failure of support for development of T cells and can be found in both mice and humans. In mice, the mutation in the nude locus results in an athymic mouse that also has no hair, the *nude mouse*. It is now known that mutation in the *whn* gene, located on the mouse chromosome 11, is responsible for abnormal development of the thymic anlage. In the *DiGeorge syndrome* in humans, an individual is born with a congenital thymic aplasia. In both conditions, only T cell development is affected as B cells

TABLE 5-1
ORIGINS OF THYMUS CELL TYPES

CELL TYPES	CELLULAR ORIGINS
Epithelium	
• Subcapsular cortex	Ectoderm of the third pharyngeal clefts
• Cortex	Endoderm of the third pharyngeal pouches
• Medulla	Ectoderm of the third pharyngeal clefts
Thymic nurse cells	Epithelium
Dendritic cells or interdigitating cells	Bone marrow
Macrophages	Bone marrow
Thymocyte	Yolk sac, fetal liver, bone marrow

develop normally. The two above conditions are also different from the *severe combined immunodeficiency syndrome (scid)*, in which the development of the thymic anlage is normal, but defects are found in the T and B cell compartments themselves.

T CELL DEVELOPMENTAL STAGES IN THE THYMUS

The *thymic anlage* provides an inductive microenvironment that allows precursor T cells to undergo rapid expansion as well as successive and distinct stages of development that can be identified by the expression of cell surface molecules. The three main differentiation cell surface molecules are CD3, CD4, CD8, and the T cell receptors (TCRs). Developing thymocytes at a specific stage of their maturation are found at a precise location within the thymus.

Precursor T cells begin to colonize the thymic anlage early during embryonic development. This begins at day 14 of embryonic age in mice and at the 7th to 8th week of gestation in humans. The rate of development of T cells within the thymus is greatest before puberty and declines sharply thereafter, although the number of mature T cells in the periphery does not show a similar reduction. The decline in the production of T cells also correlates with atrophy of the thymic stroma, a normal physiological condition known as *thymic involution*. Age-related thymic involution is known as chronic involution and is distinct from involution caused by acute infection, stress, pregnancy, and lactation. In the aging involuted thymus, one can detect changes in tissue architecture, first with increases in the volume of connective tissue and perivascular spaces and later with the replacement of the above tissues with adipose tissue. However, even in the aged individual, a small thymic rudiment composed of epithelium and thymocytes remains identifiable.

The development of monoclonal antibodies that recognize one specific epitope of a molecule greatly facilitates the characterization and identification of cells at various stages of their differentiation. Monoclonal antibodies that recognize different epitopes of the same differentiation molecule are clustered together and designated as the *cluster of differentiation (CD)* (Appendix 1).

The earliest precursor cells that arrive in the thymus lack most of the cell surface molecules that are readily detectable on mature T cells. When they arrive in the thymus, the precursor cells physically interact with thymic stromal cells, which then provide stimuli to selectively induce the expression of a group of specific cell surface molecules. In humans, the first T cell-specific molecule expressed in the thymus is CD1; in mice, CD2 and Thy-1 are expressed by the most immature T cells. These immature T cells do not express either CD4 or CD8 surface molecules and are commonly referred to as the *double negative* thymocytes. The double negative cells also do not express CD3 and thus are occasionally called the *triple negative* thymocytes. It was found recently that the earliest precursor T cells express a very low level of cell surface CD4. Thus, the most immature thymocytes in the thymus are $CD3^-CD4^{Lo}CD8^-$ that precede the double negative stage. The $CD3^-CD4^{Lo}CD8^-$ and the double negative thymocytes are found in the subcapsular cortex, where they undergo vigorous proliferation. In the next distinct stage of thymocyte maturation, thymocytes express both cell surface molecules CD4 and CD8 and are referred to as the *double positive* thymocytes; these thymocytes also begin to express the cell surface CD3 and TCR molecules. The double positive thymocyte population is the largest thymocyte population and is responsible for the dense cellularity of the thymic cortex. In contrast to the double negative cells, the double positive cells do not proliferate and are inactive. In the next stage of T cell development, the double positive cells completely cease to express either CD4 or CD8, and they mature into single positive cells that are either $CD4^+$ or $CD8^+$ (Table 5-2). The mature CD4 T cells, the *T-helper (Th) cells*, provide helper functions and cooperate with B cells in the humoral immune response, while the CD8 cells, the *cytotoxic T cells* or *CTLs*, are responsible for recognizing foreign cells, as in foreign grafts (see Chap. 17), as well as virus-infected cells and are responsible for killing these cells. Thus, as the precursor cells traverse through the subcapsular cortex, the cortex, the corticomedullary junction, and the medulla, they interact with thymic stroma and are induced to develop and mature.

TABLE 5-2
COMPARTMENTALIZATION OF α:β T CELL
DEVELOPMENTAL STAGES IN THE THYMUS

THYMIC COMPARTMENTS	THYMOCYTE SUBSETS	STATUS OF TCR GENE REARRANGEMENT	
		α	β
Subcapsular cortex	$CD3^-CD4^{Lo}CD8^-$ ↓	Germline or unrearranged	Germline or unrearranged
	$CD3^-CD4^-CD8^-$ ↓	Germline or unrearranged	Rearranged
Cortex	$CD3^+CD4^+CD8^+TCR^+$ ↓	Rearranged	Rearranged
Medulla	$CD3^+CD4^+TCR^+$ or $CD3^+CD8^+TCR^+$	Rearranged	Rearranged

PHYSICAL STRUCTURES OF T CELL RECEPTOR (TCR) GENES

At the gene level, the TCR genes α, β, γ, and δ are organized into separate gene segments designated variable (V), diversified (D), joining (J), and constant (C) regions. The α and γ genes only have the V, J, and C segments, while the β and δ genes have all four segments. There are more than one V, D, J, and C within each gene locus, with the V and J segments having the highest number; the numbers of each gene segment are different in mice and humans.

As in the case of B cells, a unique feature in T cell development is the generation of T cells, each with a specific TCR that recognizes a specific peptide antigen. While B cells recognize conformational epitopes, the TCR expressed on T cells recognizes antigenic peptides that are associated with the *major histocompatibility complex (MHC)* that are presented by antigen-presenting cells

(APC) (see Chaps. 6 and 7 for details). The generation of a large population of T cells, each cell with a unique TCR specificity, is achieved by cutting and joining regions of various gene segments encoding the TCR. The process is known as *gene rearrangement* and is executed by the products of two separate genes, the *recombination-activating genes 1 and 2 (RAG-1, RAG-2)* (Table 5-2). The end result is a collection of all specificities of TCR expressed on T cells that is termed the *T cell repertoire*.

The cell surface TCR is a heterodimer consisting of gene products from four distinct genes: α, β, γ, and δ (Fig. 5-1). The α chain of the TCR only pairs with the β chain, while the γ chain only pairs with the δ chain. This specific pairing generates two distinct subpopulations of T cells with two distinct TCRs: the most abundant population of αβ TCR T cells and the minor population of γδ TCR T cells. In mice, the appearance of γδ T cells precedes αβ T cells, and the γδ T cells and αβ T cells develop separately from the uncommitted T cell precursors. The development of γδ T cells in humans is not well characterized.

Within the αβ T cell population, the order of gene rearrangement and expression of the rearranged α and β chains on the cell surface occurs in a strictly regulated fashion, paralleling the maturation of T cells from the double negative to the double positive stage. The β chain rearranges first in the double negative cells. Since the D and J genes of the β chain are organized into two clusters of D, J, and C (see Fig. 5-1), there are two chances for a Vβ gene to join to a DJ segment in each chromosome (total of four chances to rearrange a Vβ gene in a pair of chromosomes). If a cell fails all four chances to rearrange the Vβ genes productively, it will die. Successful rearrangement of a Vβ on one chromosome also prevents the cell from continuing to rearrange a second Vβ gene; this is known as *allelic exclusion*. The successful rearrangement of the β chain with productive and functional β chain protein will ensure the expression of the single β chain on the cell surface of the double negative cells. It has been found that the β chain is expressed on the cell surface in association with a novel protein termed pre-TCR. It is possible that the β-pre-TCR complex functions as a receptor for an unknown ligand that induces expression of CD4 and CD8 and triggers the rearrangement of the TCR α chain gene. In contrast with the β chain rearrangement that complies with allelic exclusion, the V segments of the α chain (Vα) are rearranged on both chromosomes 14. In addition, the high number of the J segments (70 in humans and 50 in mice) allows more chances for a productive rearrangement of the TCR Vα genes. Because the δ locus is located within the α locus, rearrangement of the Vα genes results in deletion of the δ gene locus (see Fig. 5-1). After successful rearrangement of both α and β chains, the double positive cells now express the TCR αβ chains. At this stage, although TCR αβ are expressed on the cell surface, RAG-1 and RAG-2 genes continue to be expressed, allowing other Vα genes to rearrange. Expression of RAG-1 and RAG-2 genes is terminated only after completion of the positive selection process, discussed later in this chapter.

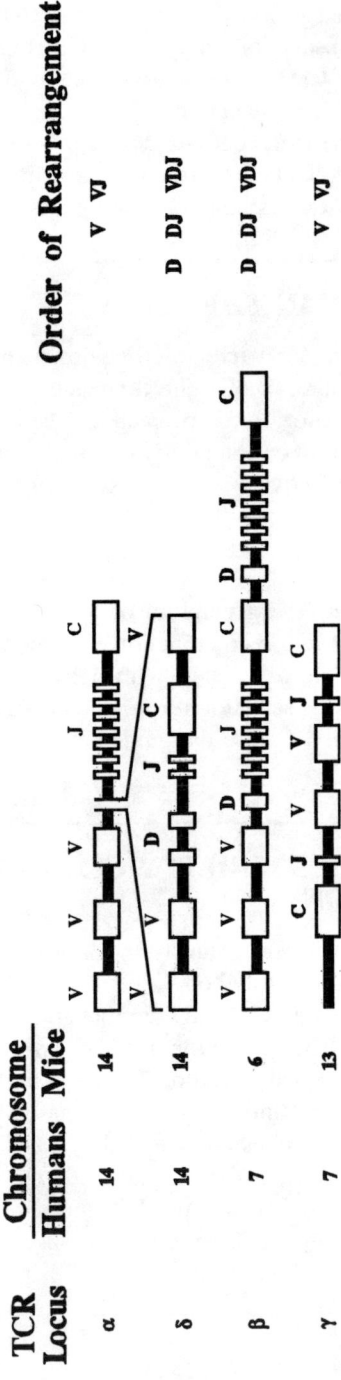

Figure 5-1

Organization of the T cell receptor α, δ, β and γ chain genes in humans and mice. In the α and γ chains, the order of rearrangement is VJ since there are no D segments. In contrast, the order of rearrangement is D to J and DJ to V forming VDJ in the β and δ T cell receptor chain genes.

The TCR $\alpha\beta$ is expressed in association with the CD3 molecule, which forms the functional signal transduction unit of the TCR (Fig. 5-2) (see Chap. 8 for details). The cell surface CD3 molecules consist of five chains: γ, δ, ϵ (epsilon), ζ (zeta), and η (eta). The ζ can either form $\zeta\zeta$ homodimers, or $\zeta\eta$ heterodimers. However, the majority of TCR is associated with the $\zeta\zeta$ homodimers as shown in Fig. 5-2. The γ and δ chains of the CD3 are different from the TCR γ and δ chains, which are only expressed on a minor population of T cells.

T CELL SELECTION IN THE THYMUS

In addition to providing an inductive microenvironment for precursor T cells to develop into mature T cells, the thymus executes two critical screening processes to select for useful, protective T cells (positive selection) and to eliminate irrelevant or potentially harmful autoreactive T cells (negative selection). Both selective processes take place at the double positive stage.

As we have just discussed, the generation of the T cell repertoire by the process of gene rearrangement and recombination is random. Since TCRs can only recognize antigenic peptide associated with MHC and presented by an antigen-presenting cell (APC), the selection for functional TCRs is dependent on the type of MHC expressed on APC. These arguments lay the foundation for the concept of *MHC restriction*.

MAJOR HISTOCOMPATIBILITY COMPLEX (MHC) RESTRICTION

It has been proven that when T cells from strain A mice are given a choice to react with foreign antigen presented on APC of strain A or B, they will preferentially react with strain A APC and therefore are restricted by MHC type A. The concept of MHC restriction further separates the antigen recognition specificity of TCR expressed on T cells from the Ig expressed by B cells, whose ability to bind antigen does not require MHC restriction.

In general, mature CD4 T cells are selected by MHC class II, while mature CD8 T cells are selected by MHC class I on the cortical thymic epithelium (see Chap. 6 for classification of MHC molecules). Thus, MHC expressed by cortical thymic epithelium dictates the specificity of the positively selected TCR.

To prove that the TCRs are selected by their ability to interact with a certain MHC type, one needs to do two things: first, to construct an individual in which

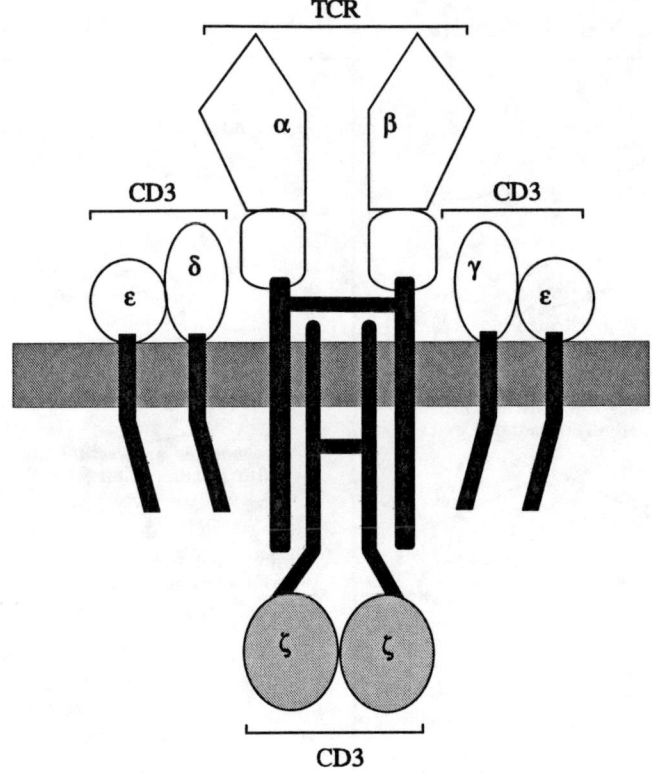

Figure 5-2
Structures of the T cell receptor-CD3 complex (TCR-CD3) expressed on the cell surface of αβ T cells. The α, β chains of the TCR form the antigenic peptide binding site, while the CD3 complex function as signal transducing components. Disulfide bonds are present between the TCR α, β chains, and between two CD3-ζ chains.

the precursor T cells and the microenvironment in which they develop, the thymic anlage, express different MHC types; and second, to develop an assay to demonstrate that the inductive environment only allows T cells with TCR specific for MHC of that thymic environment to develop. The first task is achieved by constructing *murine bone marrow chimeras*, and the second task is achieved by the successful development of the *CTL cytotoxic assay* (Fig. 5-3).

In the murine bone marrow chimeras, the precursor cells from the A×B mice are harvested from the bone marrow and are infused into either the A or B mice; each expresses the corresponding type A or B MHC. Before the cell infusion, the recipient mice are lethally irradiated (approximately 850 rad) to kill all radiation-sensitive cells, including all bone marrow-derived cells. This treatment ensures that all the bone marrow-derived cells are derived from the A×B MHC type, and this includes T cells and B cells as well as APCs. The T cells developed in the type A or B thymic environment are from the A×B precursor cells that genetically have the ability to recognize both MHC type A and MHC type B; the APCs express both MHC type A and MHC type B and are capable of presenting

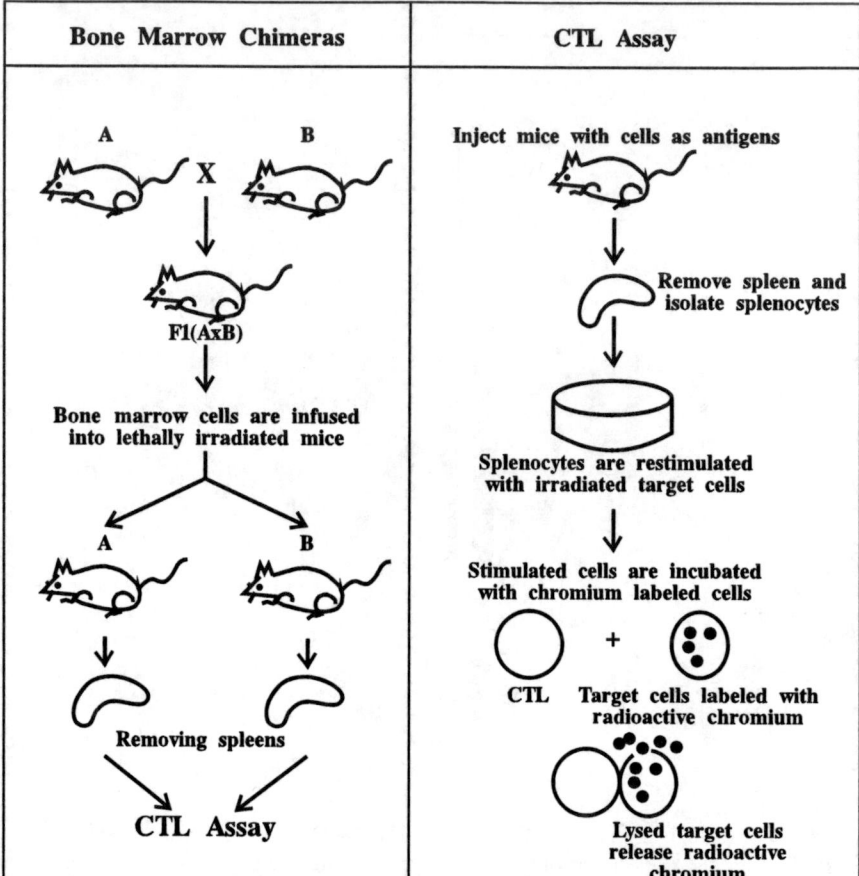

Figure 5-3

Diagram showing the constructions of bone marrow chimeras and cytotoxic T lymphocytes (CTL) assay. In the bone marrow chimeras, bone marrow cells from the F1 progeny of mouse strain A×B are used to infuse into lethally irradiated mouse strain A or B to generate the appropriate chimeras. T cells developed in the bone marrow chimeras preferentially react with either the type A or B MHC. The T cells developed in the bone marrow chimeras then can be stimulated and tested for their ability to recognize the MHC type and kill the radio-labeled target cells in the CTL assay as detailed in the right panel of the figure.

antigens to the T cells of either type A or type B MHC. Surprisingly, the MHC type of the thymic microenvironment where the T cells developed, but not the MHC type of the bone marrow precursor cells, determines the type of MHC on APC that a T cell can recognize and respond to. This means that when T cells of type A×B MHC develop in the MHC type A thymus, only the T cells with TCR that can recognize antigens presented by the MHC of the thymic stroma are selected to mature (Table 5-3). T cells with TCR that cannot recognize the MHC of the thymic stroma fail to develop and die. The thymic stroma, therefore, positively selects T cells with TCRs for MHC specificity of its own and ignores T cells with irrelevant TCR specificities. The positive selected T cells are then

TABLE 5-3
THE CTL ASSAY

In the CTL assay, the A×B precursor T cells developing in the A MHC thymic environment preferentially recognize antigens presented by the APC of the type A MHC and do not respond to antigens presented by the APC of the type B MHC. Similarly, T cells developing in a type B MHC thymic environment only respond to APC of type B and not type A MHC.

SOURCES OF BONE MARROW CELLS WITH MHC TYPES	MHC TYPE OF THE RECIPIENT THYMIC MICRO-ENVIRONMENT	CYTOTOXIC ACTIVITY OF MATURE CD8 CTL WHEN PRESENTED BY APC OF MHC TYPES	
		A	B
(A×B)F$_1$	A	++++	−
	B	−	++++
A	A	++++	−
	B	−	++++
B	A	++++	−
	B	−	++++

induced to terminate both RAG-1 and RAG-2 gene expression and to stop rearranging the TCR Vα genes. The selected T cells are committed to express the selected TCR specificity.

The developing T cells at the double positive stage also must pass a second selection process on their way to maturation. In contrast to the positive selection process in which the selected cells are supported for development, the negative selection process selectively eliminates T cells with certain TCR specificity. The negative selection process ensures that the mature T cells do not react with self-antigen presented by self-MHC. The negative selection process is best demonstrated in TCR transgenic mice with specificity for male specific antigen.

TRANSGENIC MICE

Transgenic animals have permanently incorporated exogenous genes, the *transgenes*, that are not a part of their normal genetic makeup, into their own DNA. Transgenic mice are constructed by injecting the linearized DNA containing the transgene into the male pronucleus of the fertilized eggs and subsequently implanting the fertilized eggs into pseudopregnant mice. After birth, some offspring will have incorporated the transgene and will be able to pass it on to their progeny.

TCR transgenic mice are generated by injecting both the rearranged TCR α and β chain genes into fertilized eggs and screening for offspring that express the TCR transgenes. In this experiment, the TCR genes come from a CD8 T cell that reacts with the male specific antigen known as H-Y. In the female anti-H-Y TCR transgenic mice, the β chain of the transgene is expressed on all T cells, and the endogenous β chain genes do not occur as allelic exclusion would have predicted. Since the TCR is from a CD8 clone, a higher percentage of CD8 cells mature in these transgenic mice in comparison to normal mice. In the male anti-H-Y TCR transgenic mice, all T cells with anti-H-Y TCR are deleted, and the double positive cell number is greatly reduced (Table 5-4).

Both processes of positive and negative selection effectively eliminate most T cells developed in the thymus such that greater than 90% of the developing double positive thymocytes die in the thymus. However, the intra-thymic massive cell death does not induce any chronic inflammation since these cells die by a process known as apoptosis. In the thymus, the non-selected cells or the self-reactive T cells are instructed to die by fragmenting their own DNA. With this characteristic cell death, one can detect double positive thymocytes in the thymic cortex and cortical-medullary junction that die by apoptosis due to lack of positive selection or negative selection, respectively.

TABLE 5-4
NEGATIVE SELECTION IN ANTI-H-Y TCR TRANSGENIC MICE

In the anti-H-Y TCR transgenic mice, the double positive T cells with anti-H-Y TCR that react with H-Y antigen, a self-antigen in the male, presented by APC are deleted from the double positive pool. The result is the absence of all CD8 T cells with anti-H-Y TCR specificity. In contrast to positive selection that is mediated by cortical thymic epithelium, negative selection or clonal deletion is effectively mediated by bone marrow-derived macrophages and dendritic cells.

TCR TRANSGENE	PRESENCE OF SELF-ANTIGEN	NUMBER OF DOUBLE POSITIVE THYMOCYTES
Anti-H-Y	Male: Yes	Greatly reduced
Anti-H-Y	Female: No	Normal

STRUCTURE AND ROLE OF THE MAJOR HISTOCOMPATIBILITY COMPLEX

·

- **Major Histocompatibility Complex (MHC) and Danger**
- **Genetic Organization of the MHC**
- **Structure of MHC Class I**
- **Structure of MHC Class II**
- **Immunoglobulin Supergene Family**
- **Distribution of MHC Antigens**
- **Tissue Typing**
- **HLA Disease Associations**
- **Function of the MHC**
- **MHC Restriction**

· · · · · · · · · · · ·

MAJOR HISTOCOMPATIBILITY COMPLEX (MHC) AND DANGER

The *major histocompatibility complex (MHC)* is a group of genes located on a single chromosome in all mammalian species studied so far. The MHC permits an individual who is capable of generating an immune response to distinguish *self* from what is foreign, or *non-self*.

The MHC has fundamentally evolved to provide protection from invading pathogens and virtually all substances bearing *non-self* antigens. As discussed in Chap. 5, an individual acquires the ability to distinguish self from non-self early, during T cell development and selection in the thymus. Thus, the ability to discriminate self from non-self is a T cell-dependent process. It is during T cell maturation in the thymus that T cells learn what *self* MHC is and are educated or selected to respond only to antigenic peptides presented by self MHC. Somewhat ironically, the mammalian immune system has developed to respond to *danger* to self by recognizing foreign pathogens only in the context of *self MHC*. In this way, the immune system is focused on eliminating pathogens that have become cell-associated and, therefore, pose imminent danger.

GENETIC ORGANIZATION OF THE MHC

The *human leukocyte antigen (HLA) gene complex* is the human MHC located on chromosome 6 that potentially encodes several hundred genes and is organized into three major genetic regions or loci designated class I, II, and III.

Class III genes primarily encode components of the serum complement system, which tend to be relatively conserved (i.e., nonpolymorphic) among members of the same or similar species. This group of proteins, therefore, is considered separately from MHC class I and II proteins and is discussed in Chap. 14.

Class I and II loci, on the other hand, each encode a number of highly *polymorphic* cell surface proteins, i.e., these proteins contain highly variable amino acid sequences that differ between members of the same species (Fig. 6-1). The HLA class I locus is subdivided into HLA-A, HLA-B, and HLA-C subregions, each encoding class I α chain genes. The HLA class II locus, HLA-D, is subdivided into at least six subregions (HLA-DR, -DQ, -DP, -DX, -DO, and -DZ), encoding variable numbers of α and β chain genes or pseudogenes (HLA-DO and -DZ). Despite considerable MHC polymorphism, a single individual expresses a finite number of MHC antigens and in outbred populations (i.e., humans!) is usually heterozygous for each MHC gene. This means that no single individual is capable of responding vigorously to each and every pathogen requiring a T cell response for elimination.

The ability of mammals to discriminate self from non-self was first recognized in mice that rejected tumors from mice belonging to a different strain. The ability of mice to reject foreign tissue was mapped to a region of chromosome 17 termed H-2, the mouse equivalent of the MHC. As indicated in Fig. 6-2, the arrangement of the various genetic regions of the MHC differs between species.

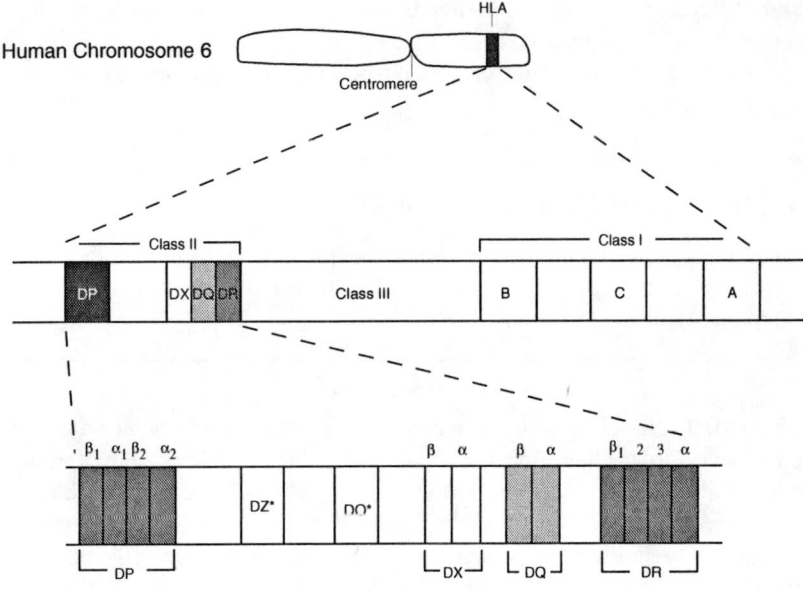

Figure 6-1
HLA gene organization.
*Pseudogenes: not expressed as protein.

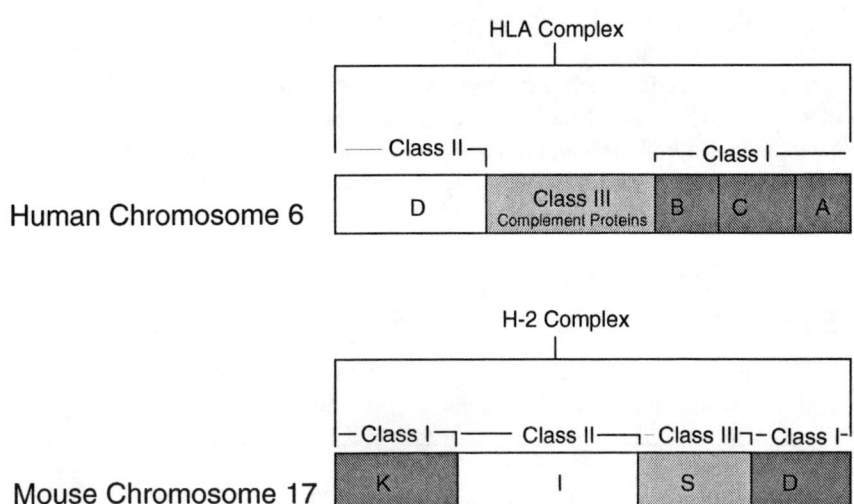

Figure 6-2
Human and mouse MHC genetic organization.

Despite different chromosomal locations, the functions of the products encoded by certain MHC loci appear to be similar, as discussed at the end of this chapter, permitting class I, II, and III designations to be made when comparing MHC from different species.

STRUCTURE OF MHC CLASS I

MHC class I is a heterodimeric molecule expressed at the cell surface that consists of two nonidentical (and therefore heterodimeric) subunits: an α chain and β_2 microglobulin.

The MHC class I molecule is a cell surface glycoprotein *heterodimer* composed of a *variable* α heavy chain (45 kd) and a nonvariable or nonpolymorphic β_2 microglobulin light chain (12-kd) (Fig. 6-3). The MHC class I α chain consists of three extracellular globular *domains*, α_1, α_2, and α_3, with the third domain, α_3 associating noncovalently with the nonpolymorphic β_2 microglobulin light chain (12 kd). β_2 microglobulin is encoded outside the MHC on chromosome 15 in the human and chromosome 2 in the mouse. Further understanding of class I structure has come from x-ray crystallographic studies, where molecules are crystallized in their purest form. These studies have indicated that α_1 and α_2 domains of the class I α heavy chain associate into a structure characterized as a *groove*. The MHC class I molecule groove consists of "sides" formed by α_1 and α_2 domain helices, as well as an interdomain "floor" consisting of a β-pleated sheet structure. Co-crystallization studies have shown that short peptide fragments of approximately nine amino acids fit into this groove. This three-dimensional MHC class I molecular conformation of α_1 and α_2 sides with a β-pleated sheet floor, therefore, represents a peptide antigen binding site, where the antigenic peptide fits the MHC molecule groove much like a baseball in a catcher's glove.

STRUCTURE OF MHC CLASS II

MHC class II is a heterodimeric molecule expressed at the cell surface that consists of two nonidentical subunits: an α chain and a β chain.

The structure of MHC class II molecules, illustrated in Fig. 6-4, is remarkably similar to class I. Although also a cell-surface glycoprotein heterodimer, the MHC class II molecule is composed of a *variable* α heavy chain (30 to 34 kd) and *variable* β light chain (26 to 29 kd). These two variable extracellular globular domains, α_1 and β_1, associate noncovalently. Recent crystallographic studies

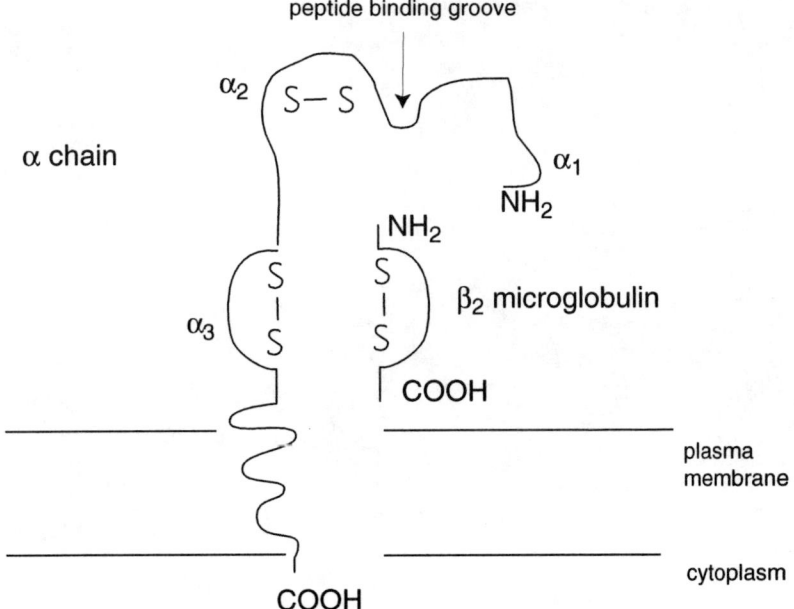

Figure 6-3
Structure of MHC class I molecule.

have indicated that, like MHC class I, class II molecules are characterized by a groove composed of helical regions of the α_1 and β_1 extracellular domains, believed to form a peptide binding site. The peptide found in the MHC class II groove is approximately 12 to 24 amino acids in length, such that the class II-antigenic peptide complex has been likened to a large peptide "frankfurter" in a smaller class II "bun."

IMMUNOGLOBULIN SUPERGENE FAMILY

This family consists of molecules such as MHC class I and II that possess immunoglobulin-like domains.

A striking characteristic of many of the cell-surface molecules that participate in the immune response is that they share remarkable structural homology. MHC molecules as well as the immunoglobulin molecule and the α and β chains of the T cell receptor all share a structural motif, namely one or more extracellular domains containing approximately 70 amino acids each. Each domain is characterized by cytosine residues, which provide a disulfide-linked closure of each domain into a globular structural unit. The immunoglobulin molecule, whose

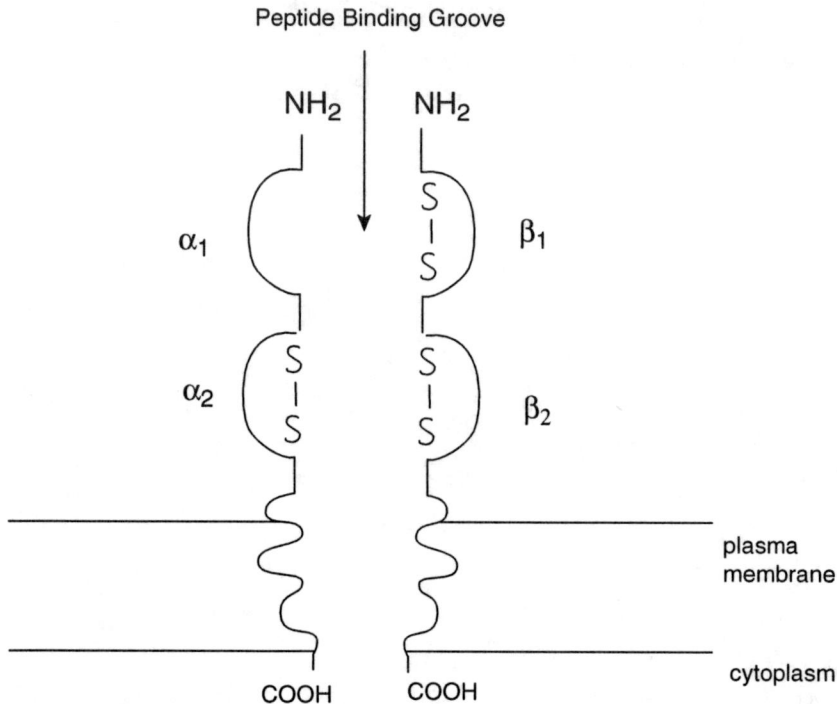

Figure 6-4
Structure of MHC class II molecule.

globular domain structure was first described, has lent its name to a group of molecules participating in various phases of the immune response, where each molecule is encoded by distinct and physically distant genes. This group of molecules is termed the *immunoglobulin supergene family* (Fig. 6-5). MHC class I and II molecules belong to this family, whose members all possess extracellular immunoglobulin-like disulfide-linked globular domains.

DISTRIBUTION OF MHC ANTIGENS

MHC molecules possess distinct patterns of tissue and cell type distribution. In general, MHC class I molecules are found on the surface of all nucleated cells. MHC class II molecules, on the other hand, are far more restricted in their distribution. B cells, macrophages, dendritic cells, and, in the human, activated T cells are among the most strongly positive for class II. Certain other cell types, notably epithelial cells, may be induced to express MHC class II during inflammatory events or in the presence of the cytokine γ interferon (Table 6-1; Appendix 2).

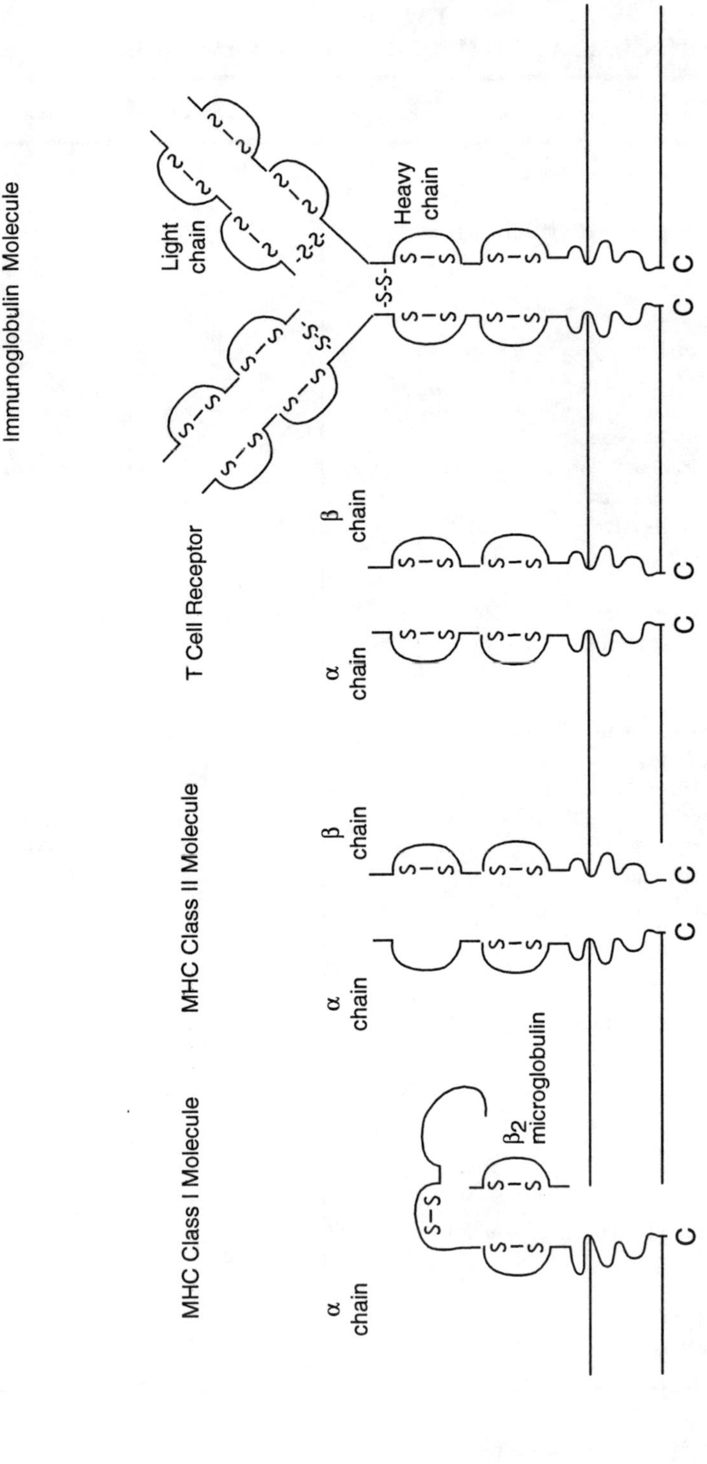

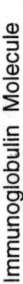

Figure 6-5
Immunoglobulin supergene family.

TABLE 6-1
MHC CLASS I AND II HUMAN TISSUE DISTRIBUTION

TISSUES	CLASS I	CLASS II
Cells of the immune system		
B cells	+ +	+ +
T cells (activated cells only)	+ +	+/−
Macrophages	+ +	+/−
Dendritic cells	+ +	+ +
Nervous system		
Peripheral	+ +	−
Central	−	−
Dura	+ +	+ +
Cardiovascular system		
Myocardium	+	−
Intercalated discs	+ +	−
Respiratory system		
Epiglottis	+ +	+ +
Trachea	+ +	+ +
Urogenital system		
Kidney glomeruli	+ +	+ +
Kidney tubules	+ +	+/−
Liver		
Sinusoidal lining cells	+ +	+ +
Hepatocytes	+/−	−
Endothelium		
Capillaries (except brain and placenta)	+ +	+ +
Larger vessels	+ +	+/−
Cells of the endocrine system		
Thyroid	+	+/−
Pituitary	+	+/−
Pancreatic Islets of Langerhans	+ +	+/−
Adrenal		−
Gastrointestinal tract (epithelium)		
Tongue	+ +	−
Esophagus	+ +	−
Stomach	+	+ +
Small intestine	+ +	−
Colon	+ +	−
Miscellaneous		
Breast (epithelial and glandular tissue)	+ +	+ +
Exocrine pancreas	−	−
Muscle	+	−
Lymphatics	+ +	+ +
Fibroblasts	+ +	−

TISSUE TYPING

Tissue typing is the identification of MHC alleles expressed on the cell surface for the purpose of matching potential tissue transplant donors and recipients.

The importance of the MHC for the success of organ transplantation became clear with early studies of tissue transplants in mice. The more MHC-identical the transplant donor and recipient, the less likely the donor transplant would be rejected and the more favorable the expected transplant outcome. Therefore, in order to optimize identity between the transplant donor and recipient, leukocytes from potential donor and recipient blood samples are examined for the identity of their MHC determinants or typed using a *cytotoxicity assay* and/or a *mixed lymphocyte reaction*. In the cytotoxicity assay, antibodies recognizing different MHC determinant specificities are applied individually to leukocytes together with complement. If the leukocyte bears an MHC molecule recognized by an anti-MHC antibody, then complement will be activated by antibody bound to the leukocyte and lysis of the cell will occur. Alternatively, in the mixed lymphocyte reaction, T cells to be tested for MHC identity are placed in culture individually with cells of known MHC identities that do not divide under the culture conditions. T lymphocytes are stimulated to proliferate in the presence of cells bearing *foreign* MHC determinants but usually do not proliferate in the presence of *self* MHC. These early studies conducted with mice were later confirmed in human studies.

HLA DISEASE ASSOCIATIONS

With the advent of human MHC or HLA typing, certain disease associations have emerged that correlate with certain HLA types. These diseases are generally autoimmune (anti-self) in nature, and a brief list of these associations is presented in Table 6-2. The exact mechanism by which certain MHC genes predispose to autoimmune disease is not yet well understood but is treated in more detail in Chap. 16.

TABLE 6-2
HLA DISEASE ASSOCIATIONS

DISEASE	ASSOCIATED HLA ANTIGEN
Myasthenia gravis	B8,DR3
Systemic lupus erythematosus	DR3
Ankylosing spondylitis	B27
Reiter's syndrome	B27
Subacute thyroiditis	B35
Psoriasis	Cw6
Celiac disease	DR3
Addison's disease	DR3
Juvenile-onset diabetes	DR3
Rheumatoid arthritis	DR4

FUNCTION OF THE MHC

- To ensure that antigen is presented by cell surface MHC molecules so that free antigen alone does not saturate T cell receptor (TCR) molecules, thus preventing elimination of danger to cells.
- To ensure, by diversifying MHC across a species (*MHC polymorphism*), that the species as a whole may respond to antigen and survive danger, since a single MHC molecule is incapable of binding to and presenting all antigens.

Insight into the function of MHC molecules was obtained with the demonstration that cytotoxic or killer T cells isolated from a mouse that had been immunized with a virus could only recognize and destroy virally infected cells from the same or MHC-identical mouse strain (MHC-restriction). These cytotoxic cells could not recognize and destroy cells from an MHC nonidentical mouse strain infected with the same virus (Fig. 6-6). Thus, the immune response has come to be known as being self *MHC-restricted*. Not only does the MHC appear to function in the context of defining what is *self*, but the immune response is restricted to participation within an environment defined as *self*. Such commitment to self occurs early during development and requires the thymus (see Chap. 5) to create and monitor the MHC-restricted environment of the adaptive immune system. In this way, the MHC is absolutely required for self-recognition and the induction of an effective T cell-dependent immune response during antigen processing and presentation (see Chap. 7).

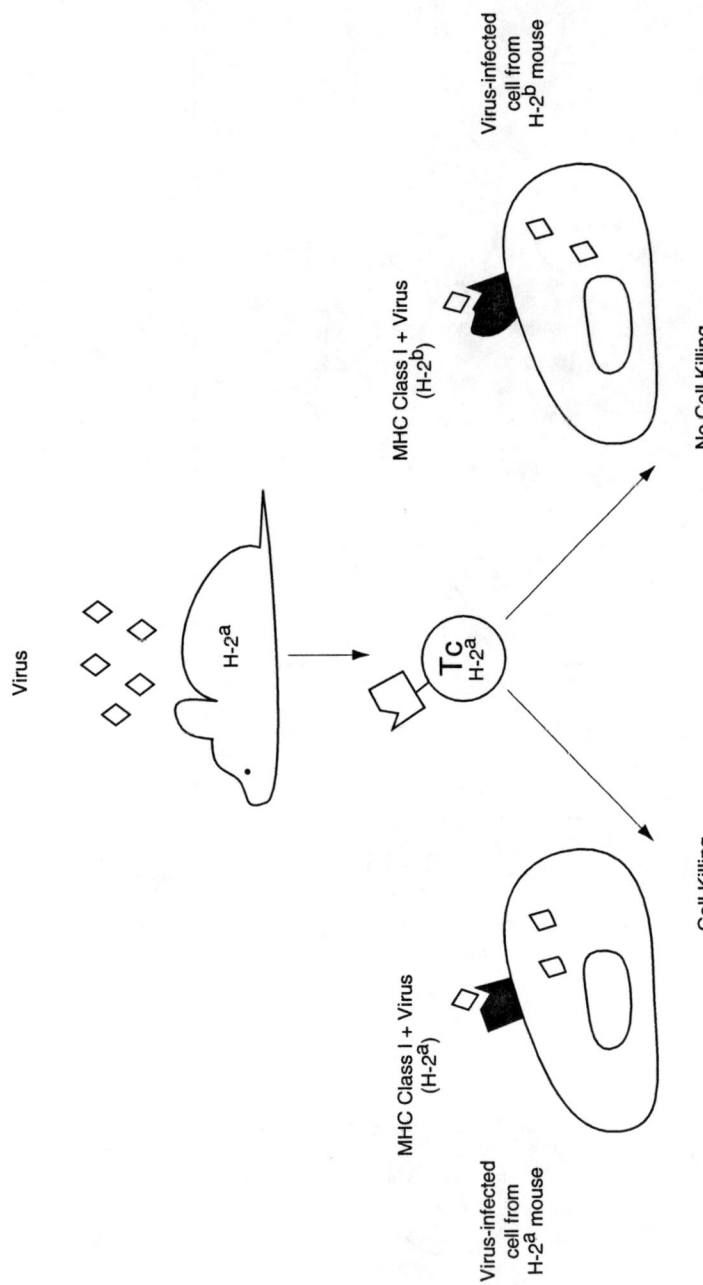

Figure 6-6
MHC restriction of cytotoxic T cell killing.

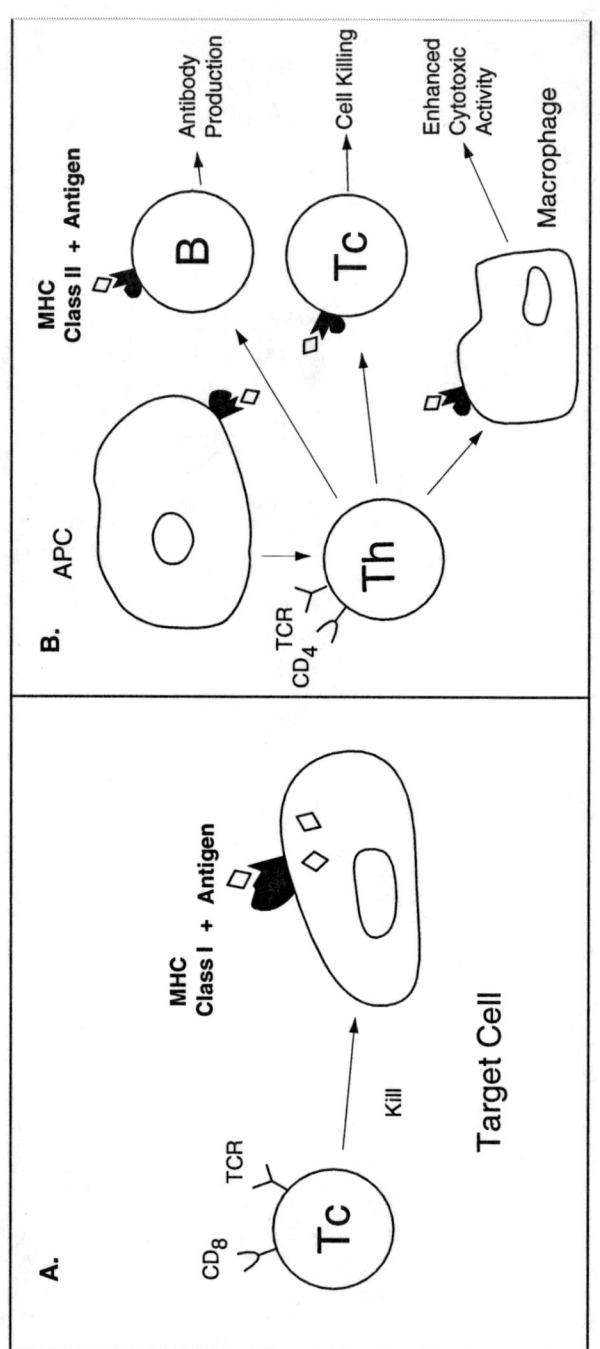

A. Direct Cell Killing

B. T-dependent Help

Figure 6-7
Functions of the MHC.

MHC RESTRICTION

MHC class I
Located on the surface of all nucleated cells
Presents peptides derived from endogenous antigens
Recognized by CD8+ cells

MHC class II
Located on B cells, macrophages, dendritic cells, and activated T cells
Presents peptides derived from exogenous antigens
Recognized by CD4+ T cells

CD8+ T cells, which are usually cytotoxic cells when appropriately activated, recognize endogenous or intracellular peptide antigen only in association with or loaded into the groove of *MHC class I* molecules on target cells (Fig. 6-7A). *CD4+* T cells, which are referred to as T helper cells, are restricted to the recognition of exogenous or extracellular peptide antigen associated with *MHC class II* molecules on antigen-presenting cells (Figure 6-7B). A discussion of antigen presentation follows in Chap. 7.

The MHC has been defined as a cluster or complex of genes encoding, among other products, highly polymorphic cell surface glycoproteins. These molecules appear to be required for an effective mammalian immune response. These features may appear puzzling at first but might be explained by the following considerations. First, the high degree of polymorphism of MHC class I and II molecules concentrated at the peptide-binding region ensures that an entire species has the potential to effectively respond to and eliminate any antigen it encounters. Second, the need for an associated recognition system by the TCR in order to produce an immune response, namely antigenic peptides in association with MHC molecules, may effectively prevent saturation of the TCR with free antigen. Such a situation might otherwise prevent effective T cell help and/or killing of antigen-expressing (i.e., endangered) target cells.

ANTIGEN PROCESSING AND PRESENTATION
PART A: ANTIGEN PROCESSING

•

- **Binding and Uptake of Antigen**
- **Low Levels of Particulate or Soluble Antigens**
- **High Levels of Particulate or Soluble Antigens**
- **Viral Proteins or Tumor Proteins That Are Produced Intracellularly**
- **Antigen Processing**
- **MHC Class I Processing Pathway**
- **TAP (Transporter Associated with Antigen Processing)**
- **Calnexin**
- **Brefeldin A**
- **MHC Class II Processing Pathway**
- **Invariant Chain**
- **Chloroquine**
- **Antigenic Peptide-MHC Interaction**

• • • • • • • • • • • •

To maintain survival of the organism, cells of the immune system must be able to recognize and eliminate antigens that enter the body. Antigens that do not easily enter the cell, such as bacteria or large proteins, are recognized by cells called *antigen-presenting cells*, such as macrophages or B lymphocytes. These cells are called antigen-presenting cells because they internalize antigen and process it for presentation to specific receptors associated with CD4+ T lymphocytes. In contrast, antigens that gain entry into the cell to reside within the cell, such as viruses, are processed by the host cell for presentation to specific receptors associated with CD8+ T lymphocytes. The antigen is presented as a short peptide sequence in association with a cell surface protein encoded within the major histocompatibility complex (MHC) of the antigen-presenting cell. Thus, MHC molecules provide for the extracellular presentation of antigenic peptides that have been internalized and processed within the intracellular environment.

BINDING AND UPTAKE OF ANTIGEN

Binding and uptake of antigen into the cell depends on the physical state of the antigen and the cell type involved.

LOW LEVELS OF PARTICULATE OR SOLUBLE ANTIGENS

Low levels of antigen bind to a specific immunoglobulin receptor expressed on B cells and are internalized by a process known as endocytosis.

Also, antigens may bind to their specific receptor on an immunoglobulin that is attached to a macrophage by receptors for the Fc portion of that immunoglobulin (described in detail in Chap. 3). In this manner, the Fc receptor-bound immunoglobulin captures the antigen, and the antigen-immunoglobulin-Fc receptor complex is endocytosed. These antigens will associate with MHC class II molecules after processing.

HIGH LEVELS OF PARTICULATE OR SOLUBLE ANTIGENS

High levels of antigen are nonspecifically engulfed by macrophages by a process known as phagocytosis. These antigens will associate with MHC class II molecules after processing.

VIRAL PROTEINS OR TUMOR PROTEINS THAT ARE PRODUCED INTRACELLULARLY

These antigens escape binding and uptake by B cells and macrophages. The large proteins produced by viruses or tumors will be degraded by any somatic cell intracytoplasmically into smaller peptides and will associate with MHC class I molecules.

Extracellular antigens taken up by phagocytosis or endocytosis go directly to endosomes and/or lysosomes for antigen degradation and loading onto MHC class II molecules. Endosomal and/or lysosomal enzymes break down the protein into peptide fragments containing a short amino acid sequence. Newly synthesized MHC class II molecules will eventually be transported from the endoplasmic reticulum (ER) to the endosome/lysosome compartment, where they will associate with peptide fragments derived from extracellular antigens. On the other hand, intracellular antigenic proteins are processed into small peptides in proteosomes that contain proteases. These peptides will complex with transporter proteins that will move them to the ER to interact with newly synthesized MHC Class I molecules (Fig. 7-1).

ANTIGEN PROCESSING

Antigen processing involves the degradation of externally- or internally-derived antigen into short peptide sequences and the association of the peptide with MHC molecules. Two distinct classes of MHC molecules, MHC class I and MHC class II, regulate the presentation of antigens to either CD8+ or CD4+ cells, respectively.

The location of antigen, extracellular or intracellular, determines which MHC molecule will bind the peptide. Peptides derived from antigenic proteins that reside within the cell, such as viral proteins, bind to MHC class I molecules, while peptides derived from antigenic proteins that initially reside outside of the cell, such as either bacterial proteins or large proteins attached to small haptens (Chap. 3), bind to MHC class II molecules.

MHC CLASS I PROCESSING PATHWAY

Antigenic protein → proteosome → peptide fragment released into cytosol → binds to TAP protein → moves to ER
Newly synthesized Class I α chain and β_2 microglobulin → move to ER → calnexin binds to α chain → peptide fragment and β_2 microglobulin bind to alpha chain → release of α chain from calnexin → complex moves to Golgi apparatus → glycosylation in Golgi apparatus → secretory vesicle → plasma membrane

---

As shown in Fig. 7-1, newly synthesized nascent alpha chain and beta-2-microglobulin of the Class I MHC molecule are synthesized and translocated by ribosomes to the endoplasmic reticulum (ER) where they interact with not only each other, but also with processed antigenic peptide fragments released from proteosomes.

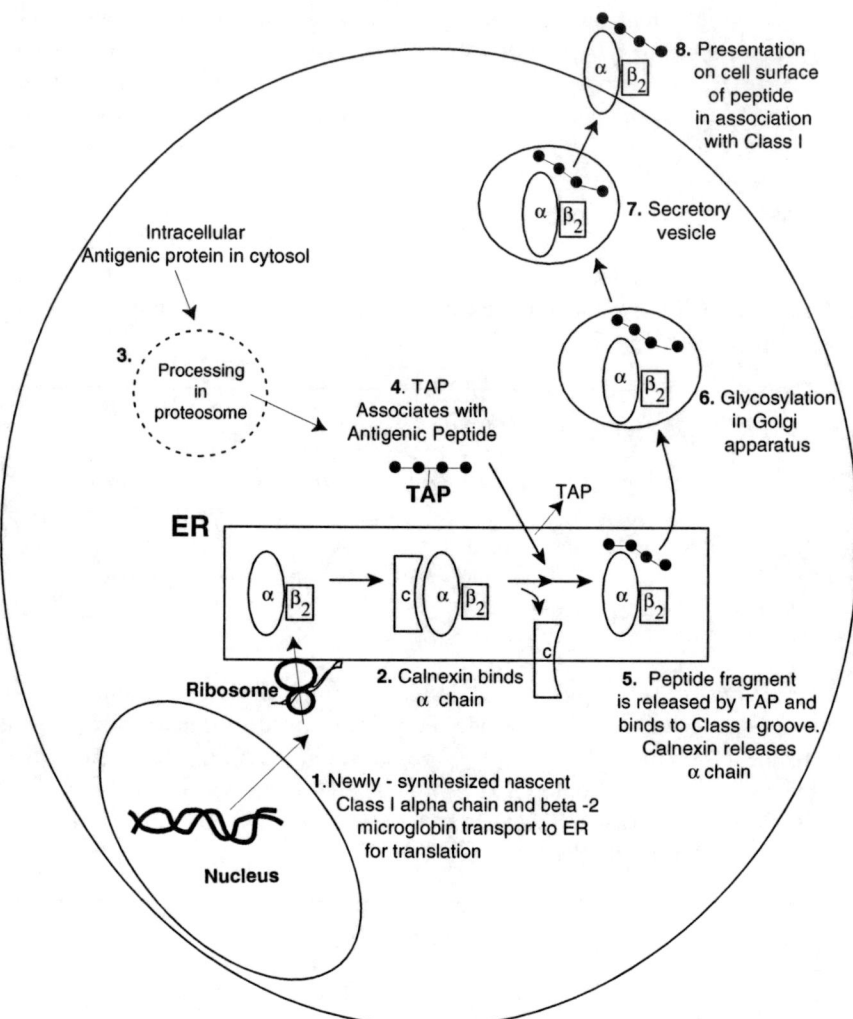

Figure 7-1
MHC class I processing pathway.

TAP (TRANSPORTER ASSOCIATED WITH ANTIGEN PROCESSING

TAP is a protein that transports small peptides in the cytosol to the ER so that they can be loaded onto MHC class I molecules.

In order for small antigenic peptides located in the cytosol to become attached to class I molecules, they must be transported from the cytosol to the ER by a transporter protein, TAP, which is specific for peptide size and amino acid sequence. In this manner, TAP binding of small antigenic peptides excludes the possibility of class I molecules binding to large unprocessed proteins. From the ER, the class I molecule-antigenic peptide complex passes through the Golgi, where *glycosylation* occurs before export of the complex to the cell surface.

CALNEXIN

Calnexin is an 88-kd integral ER membrane chaperone protein that binds to a nascent MHC class I α chain after release from a ribosome into the ER lumen so that the α chain will not leave the ER until it binds both a short peptide sequence and β_2 microglobulin.

Class I molecules in the ER that are waiting to bind peptides are retained in the ER by the binding of calnexin to the α chain. In order for class I molecules to move from the ER to the Golgi, calnexin must dissociate from the α chain. This dissociation of calnexin from the α chain requires that both the short peptide sequence and β_2 microglobulin bind to the α chain. Upon dissociation from calnexin, the α chain-β_2 microglobulin-peptide complex is transported to and through the Golgi apparatus for glycosylation and then into a secretory vesicle that moves to the outside of the plasma membrane. The result of this process of checks and balances is that no free MHC class I is present on the cell surface to bind exogenous antigens. In this manner, the T cell receptor of a CD8+ cell focuses on cells that are actively infected and, thus, express an antigenic peptide of that infectious intracellular agent in the groove of their MHC class I.

BREFELDIN A

Brefeldin A is a drug that specifically blocks the passage of the MHC class I-antigenic peptide complex through the Golgi apparatus, resulting in no MHC class I-peptide complex expressed on the cell surface.

If this drug is present, MHC class I-antigenic peptide complexes will accumulate intracellularly and will not be detected on the cell surface. This will show that movement of the complexes through, and the glycosylation of the complexes within, the Golgi complex are essential for the packaging of the complexes into secretory vesicles for delivery to the cell surface.

MHC CLASS II PROCESSING PATHWAY

Antigenic protein → endosome/lysosome → peptide fragment
Newly synthesized class II molecules → move to ER and associate with
   invariant chain protein molecule → move to Golgi apparatus → move
   to endosomes/lysosomes → release of invariant chain from class II
   molecule → class II binds antigenic peptide fragment → transport to
   cell surface

In contrast to class I molecules, as shown in Fig. 7-2, MHC class II molecules associate with antigenic peptide fragments that are derived from exogenous antigens that have been endocytosed into endosomes/lysosomes that reside within the cytosol. Newly synthesized class II molecules are transported to the ER and then directly to the Golgi apparatus. From the Golgi, class II molecules move into either endosomes or lysosomes, where they bind peptide fragments, as opposed to binding peptide fragments in the ER as occurs for class I molecules. A molecule that helps in the orchestration of this specific transport of class II molecules to the endosomes/lysosomes for binding of the peptide fragment is called the *invariant chain*.

INVARIANT CHAIN

The invariant chain directs the movement of newly synthesized class II molecules into the Golgi and then the late endocytic compartment of the cell.

Invariant chain also prevents the binding of antigenic peptides to class II molecules, at least until the class II molecule reaches the late endocytic compartment, a location where antigenic peptides and class II molecules bind together for the first time.

It is still a point of debate as to the exact location of peptide loading onto class II molecules, but most data show that loading occurs within either a late endosome or a lysosome where the environment becomes increasingly more acidic. Thus, a combination of acidic pH and proteases within the endosome/lysosome cleaves the invariant chain from the class II molecule and exposes the peptide binding site. The MHC class II molecule-antigenic peptide complex then moves to the cell surface.

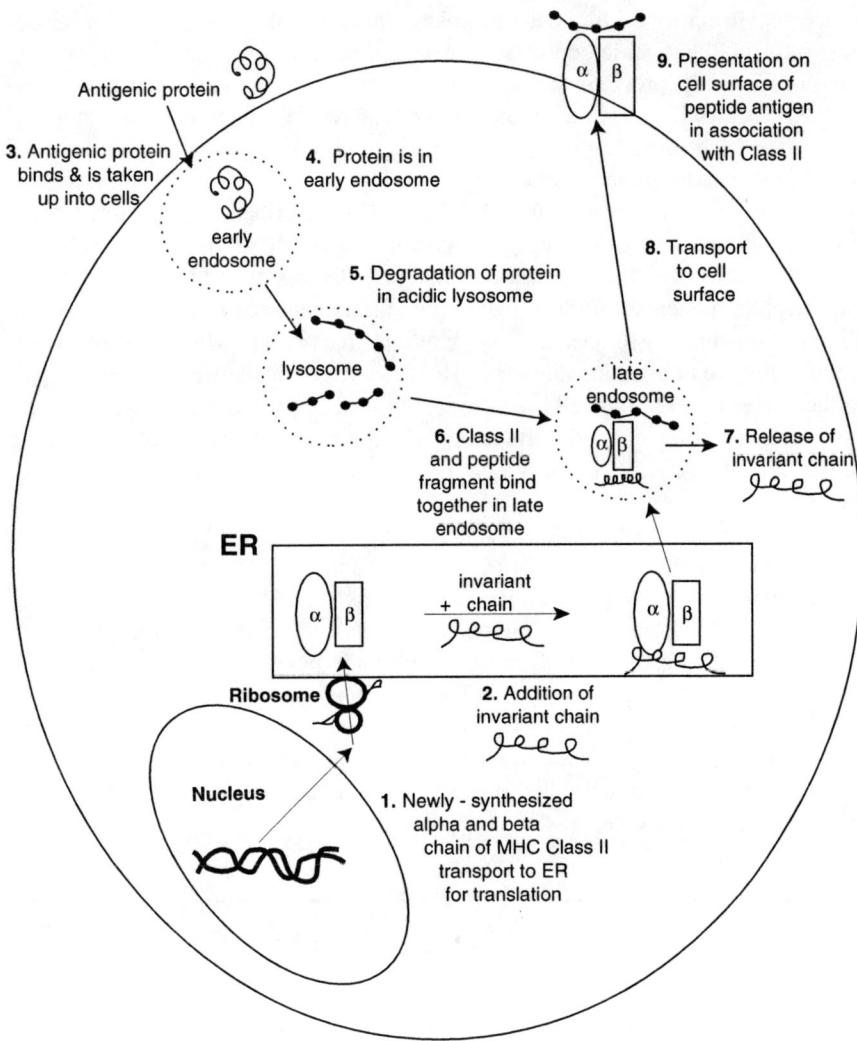

Figure 7-2
MHC class II processing pathway.

CHLOROQUINE

Chloroquine is a drug that effectively raises the pH of early endosomes and lysosomes, thus making the environment more basic.

A basic environment within these compartments prevents the degradation of proteins into small antigenic peptides. Use of this drug prevents antigen processing and, consequently, prevents the production of antigenic peptides that would complex MHC class II molecules in the late endosome. This is an experimental tool that is used to show that antigen processing is required in order to obtain an MHC class II-restricted immune response.

The structure and role of the MHC have been desribed in detail in Chap. 6. Analysis of these molecules by X-ray crystallography shows that each HLA gene encodes regions of the intact molecule that provide a peptide binding groove for short peptide sequences of the antigen. The variable nature of the MHC molecule is localized primarily to these peptide binding grooves, allowing the host to present a multitude of invading antigens. All MHC molecules on the surface of a particular antigen-presenting cell bind the same linear sequence of amino acids from the processed antigen. In this manner, all of the peptide-MHC complexes on the surface of one APC are only able to associate with a single T cell receptor specificity.

The length of the peptide sequence in association with MHC molecules is critical, since the shorter the peptide length of antigen, the more likely it is that proteins normally present within the cell will also contain the same sequence of amino acids. This possibility means that immune cells might recognize self proteins and react against them. Therefore, antigenic peptides must be of a length that ensures their recognition by the T cell receptor as antigenic but not as self. However, it should be noted, as described in detail in Chap. 5, that short amino acid sequences that are generated from host self proteins will have already been presented to self-reactive T cells to inactivate them during development of the T cell repertoire in the thymus.

ANTIGENIC PEPTIDE-MHC INTERACTION

Peptides that bind to MHC class I grooves are usually between 8 and 10 amino acids in length, while peptides that bind to MHC class II grooves are usually between 12 and 24 amino acids. The peptide sequence binds tightly to the MHC molecule at several points so that recognition by the T cell receptor can occur before the peptide dissociates from the MHC molecule.

The requirement for a short peptide sequence to bind to MHC molecules means that most protein antigens must be broken down into smaller peptides to destroy the secondary and tertiary structure of large protein antigens. Some protein antigens, such as foreign insulin, require limited breakdown to expose the antigenic epitope needed to bind to the MHC molecule, while others, such as foreign fibrinogen, require no breakdown.

PART B: ANTIGEN PRESENTATION

•

- **Antigen Presentation to T Cells**
- **Associated Recognition of Antigenic Peptide and MHC**
- **Superantigens**
- **Antigen-presenting Cells**

•   •   •   •   •   •   •   •   •   •   •   •

ANTIGEN PRESENTATION TO T CELLS

Antigen presentation is, strictly speaking, the activation of T cells via T cell receptors, which specifically recognize antigenic peptide in association with either MHC class I or II molecules on the surface of antigen-presenting cells (APCs).

The discussion of the MHC in Chap. 6 and of the requirements for *antigen processing* previously in this chapter emphasizes the fact that T cells effectively respond to most foreign antigens in the context of antigenic peptide plus MHC. At this point, it is worth noting that B cells are capable of recognizing and binding certain antigens without MHC restriction by virtue of their cell surface antigen receptor, the immunoglobulin or antibody molecule.

For the purposes of this discussion, we will concentrate on the T cell as the primary cell responding to antigen presentation. T cells recognize antigen only in the context of appropriate (i.e., self) MHC molecules (Fig. 7-3). Self MHC is

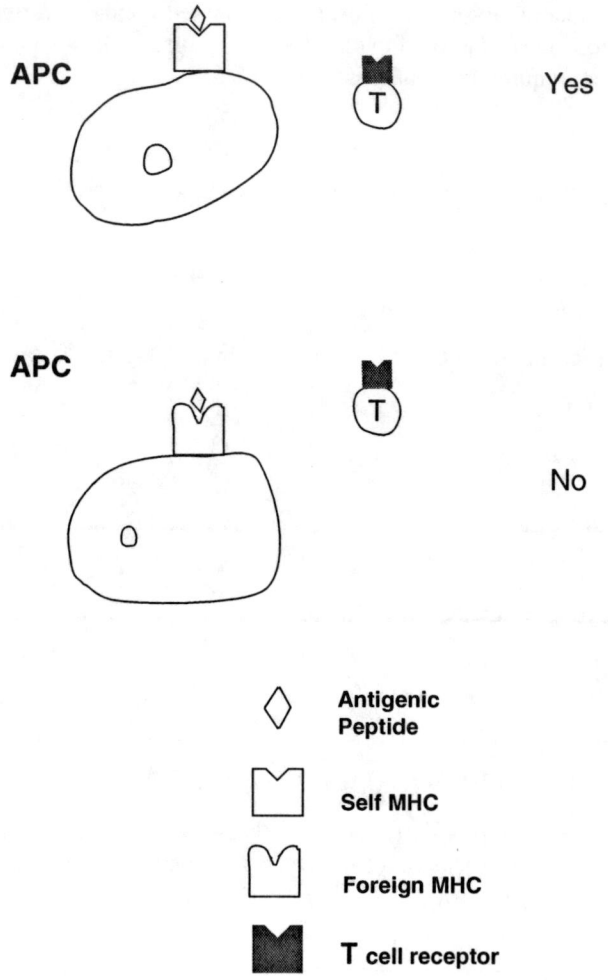

Figure 7-3
Antigen presentation.

therefore required for effective antigen presentation to T cells, which are activated to offer T cell help or cytotoxic activity. As mentioned in Chap. 6, CD8$^+$ T cells, usually cytotoxic, recognize antigen only in association with MHC class I molecules. CD4$^+$ T cells, usually T-helper cells, are restricted to recognizing antigen only in association with MHC class II molecules.

ASSOCIATED RECOGNITION OF ANTIGENIC PEPTIDE AND MHC

Two theories may explain the requirement that a T cell-dependent antigen be presented together with MHC antigens in order to generate an effective immune response. According to the *dual recognition* theory, a T cell might bear two distinct receptors, one receptor binding to antigenic peptide and the other binding to MHC molecules. The other theory, that of *associated recognition*, requires that the T cell bear one receptor capable of binding both antigenic peptide and MHC molecules.

The two theories of recognition illustrated in Fig. 7-4, have been tested. Imagine a "hybrid" T cell resulting from the fusion of one parental T cell of a defined antigen (A) and MHC (k) specificities with a T cell bearing different antigen (B) and MHC (l) specificities. The associated recognition theory argues that such a T cell hybrid would only respond to or proliferate in response to the original parental antigen-MHC specificities. (A^k or B^l) but *not* A^l or B^k.

If, on the other hand, *dual recognition* of antigen and MHC molecules by two distinct receptors on T cells were operative, such a hybrid T cell should respond to all four antigen-MHC specificities: A^k, B^l, A^l, and B^k, due to independent association of T cell antigen and MHC receptors. Such responses were not found when T cell hybrids were tested. All experimental evidence has thus far supported the *associated recognition theory* of antigen and MHC by T cells. We now know that a single T cell receptor recognizes both MHC and antigen specificities. More recently, detailed knowledge of both the structure of the MHC molecule and its own capacity to bind peptide antigen, discussed in Chap. 6, has refined our understanding of T cell antigen recognition. Depicted in Fig. 7-5 is a more accurate interpretation of TCR binding to both antigen and MHC molecules, class I in the case of $CD8^+$ T cells and class II in the case of $CD4^+$ T cells. As the T cell receptor (TCR) engages with the antigenic peptide-MHC molecule complex, T cell CD4 molecules bind to a conserved region of the MHC class II molecule, and CD8 molecules bind a conserved region of the MHC class I molecule.

SUPERANTIGENS

Superantigens are certain bacterial and viral glycoproteins that bind TCR and MHC class II antigens outside of the conventional groove for antigenic peptide binding, leading to nonspecific activation of multiple T cell clones.

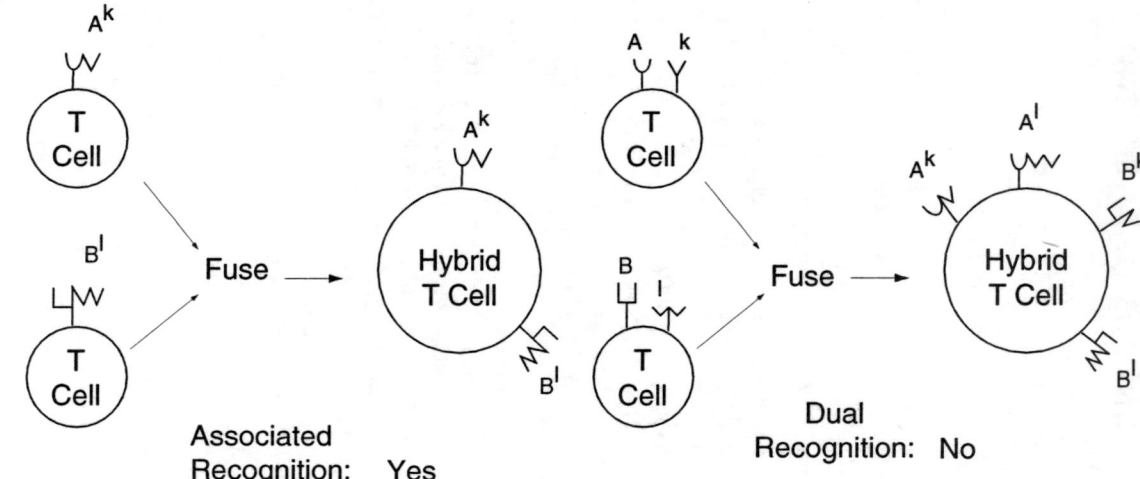

Associated Recognition: Yes

Dual Recognition: No

A, B = antigen receptor specificity
k, l = MHC receptor specificity

Figure 7-4
Associated vs. dual antigen recognition by T cells.

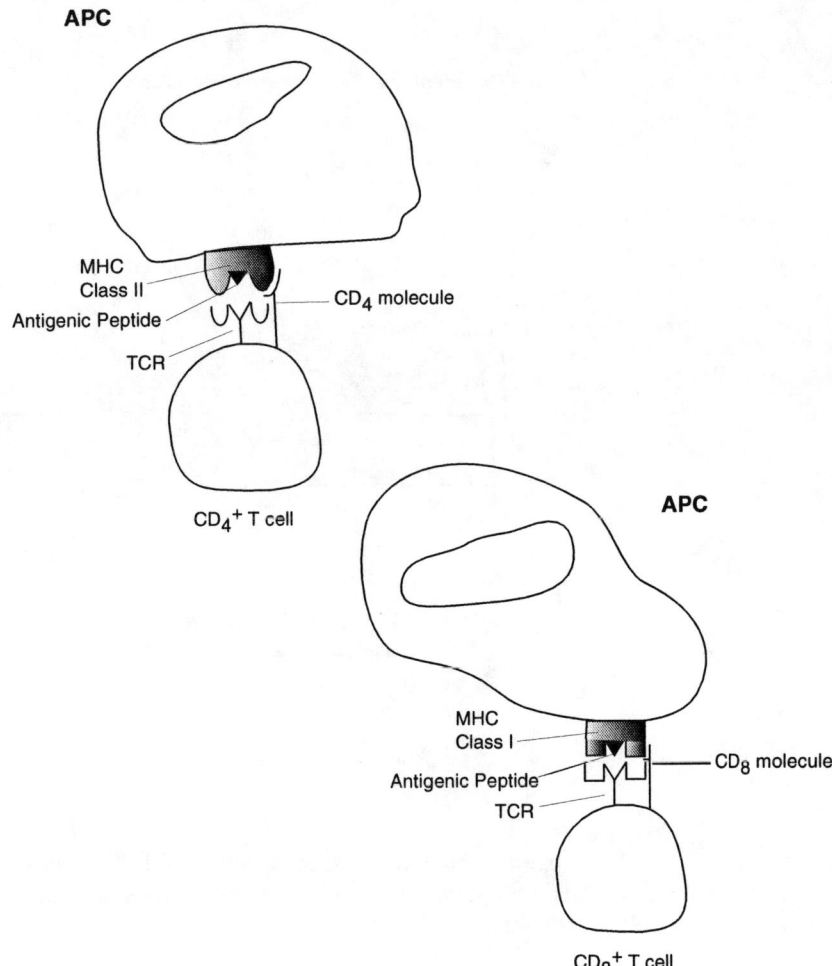

Figure 7-5
Antigen recognition by T cells.

While a single peptide antigen may be recognized by or is immunogenic for a small number of T cell clones, a special category of antigens, known as *super-antigens*, have the capacity to stimulate multiple T cell clones. Superantigens, which have been identified thus far as bacterial and viral glycoproteins, are *super-stimulators* of T cells because they are capable of binding to a large number of T cell receptor Vβ sequences, as well as to MHC class II molecules outside of the peptide presentation groove. As illustrated in Fig. 7-6, the binding of superanti-gens to relatively nonpolymorphic regions of MHC and TCR molecules promotes

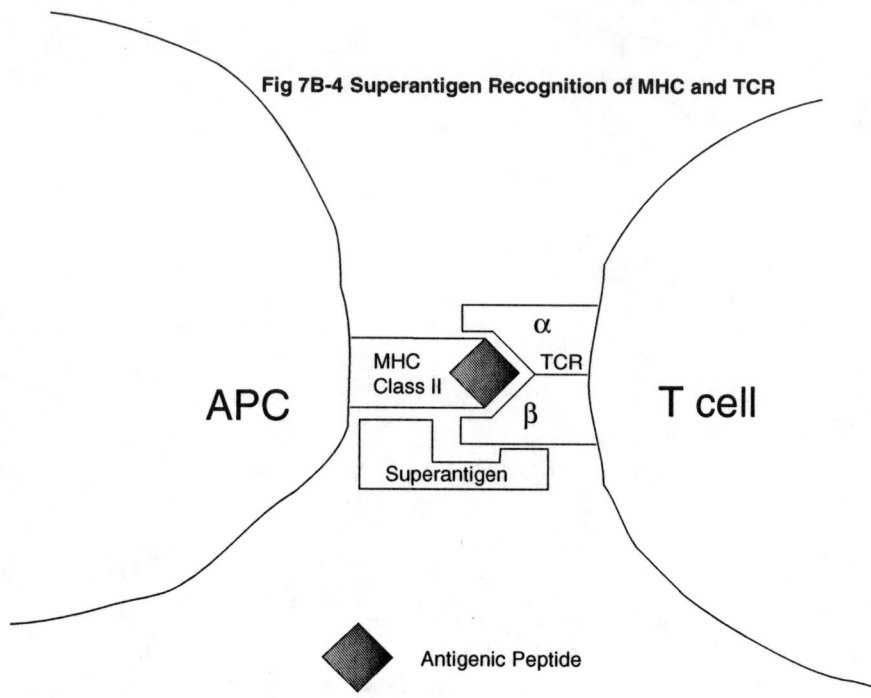

Figure 7-6
Superantigen recognition of MHC and TCR.

adherence of T cells to antigen-presenting cells, irrespective of TCR specificity. Such cross-linking of TCR with MHC molecules leads to the activation of multiple clones of T cells, especially CD4$^+$ cells.

ANTIGEN-PRESENTING CELLS

Macrophages, dendritic cells, B cells, and virtually any other cell type capable of expressing MHC class II molecules may function as *antigen-presenting cells* (*APCs*) (Table 7-1). Recall that CD4+ T-helper cells recognize and respond to antigen in the context of MHC class II.

Macrophages are phagocytic cells of the monocytic lineage residing within tissues and are particularly well equipped for effective antigen presentation. They

TABLE 7-1
ANTIGEN-PRESENTING CELLS

APC	PRESENT TO
Macrophages	T cells via MHC antigens
Dendritic cells	T cells via MHC antigens
B cells	T cells via antigen capture by surface antibody and MHC antigens
Activated T helper cells	T cells via MHC antigens

generally express MHC class II molecules and along with their phagocytic properties are extremely efficient at engulfing macromolecular or particulate material, digesting it, processing it with an extensive lysosomal system to antigenic peptide form, and expressing it on the cell surface for recognition by T lymphocytes.

Dendritic cells, so named for their highly branched morphology, are found in many organs throughout the body, are bone marrow-derived and usually express high levels of MHC class II antigen. Dendritic cells are actively motile and can recirculate between the bloodstream and tissues. Unlike macrophages, dendritic cells possess a limited capacity for antigen processing and may present antigen previously processed and released from other cells. In this way, they too are considered important APCs. Langerhans cells are an example of dendritic cells that are located in the skin.

B lymphocytes, as discussed in Chapter 4, while not actively phagocytic, are class II-positive and possess cell surface antigen-specific receptors, immunoglobulin, or antibody molecules. Due to their potential for high affinity antigen binding, B cells are uniquely endowed with the capacity to concentrate low concentrations of antigen on their surface, endocytose it, process it, and present it in the context of antigenic peptide in association with MHC antigen on their surface. In this manner, B cells become extremely effective APCs.

While not considered classic APCs, T-helper cells deserve mention for their capacity to act as such under certain conditions of T-helper cell activation. In humans and other mammalian species, with the exception of the mouse, activated T cells are induced to express MHC class II molecules and also to up-regulate MHC class I. Such activation events may serve to recruit additional CD4+ T cell help for B cells as well as to offer effective T cell help to the CD8+ T cytotoxic cell.

A simplified overview of antigen processing and presentation is presented in Fig. 7-7.

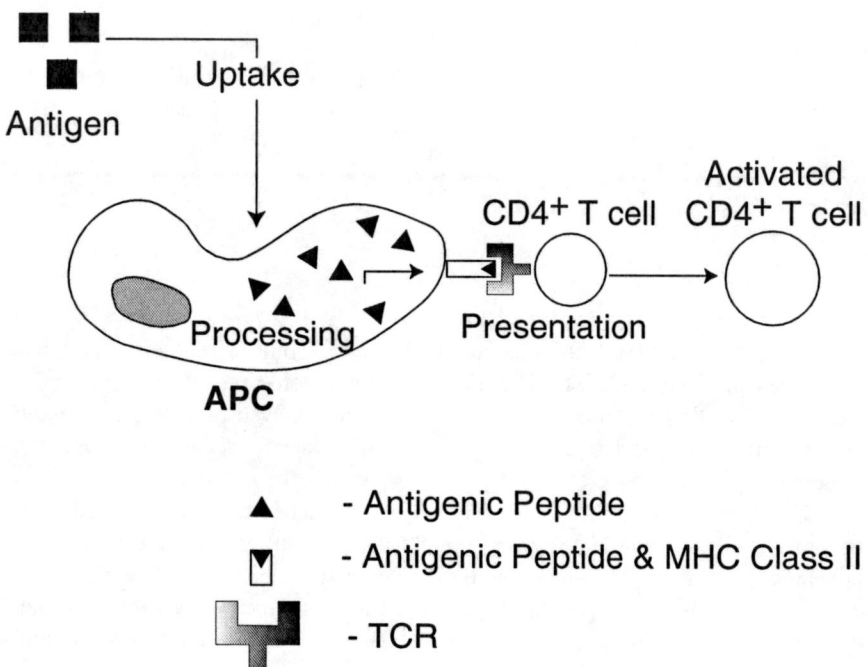

Figure 7-7
Antigen processing and presentation.

T CELL RECEPTOR: STRUCTURES AND FUNCTIONS IN T CELL ACTIVATION

·

- **Anatomical Structure of the T Cell Receptor (TCR)**

- **Superantigens**

- **CD3 Molecules as a Component of the TCR Complex**

- **Signal-transducing Components of the CD3-TCR Complex**

- **CD4 and CD8 Co-receptors**

- **T Cell Activation**

· · · · · · · · · · · ·

As in B cells that synthesize immunoglobulins (Igs) with specificity for antigens (see Chap. 4), T cells express receptors (*T cell receptors*, *TCRs*) that specifically bind to antigenic peptides. Each mature T cell expresses approximately 30,000 TCRs. Although both B cell-derived Igs and TCRs can recognize and bind to antigens, there are several important salient features that distinguish TCRs from Igs. First, the TCR is an integral cell membrane molecule and is not a secretory product like certain Igs. Second, the secreted bivalent IgG binds to soluble antigens; TCR is monovalent and can only recognize and bind to antigenic peptides when these peptides are incorporated into the groove of the MHC class I or class II and the antigen-MHC complexes presented by an antigen-presenting cell (APC) (see Chaps. 6 and 7). The TCR complex has *two distinct molecules*: the *TCR*, which binds antigen-MHC, and the *CD3* molecules, which function as the signal-transducing components. Expression of both CD3 and TCR is required for activating T cells and generating effector T cells. In this chapter we will discuss the anatomical structures of the TCR-CD3 receptor complex, how TCR binds to the antigen-MHC complex, how T cells are activated because of this binding, and the cellular and molecular events following the activation of T cells.

ANATOMICAL STRUCTURE OF THE T CELL RECEPTOR (TCR)

TCR is a heterodimer comprising $\alpha\beta$ chains or $\gamma\delta$ chains. Most peripheral T cells in secondary lymphoid organs such as spleen and lymph nodes express the TCR $\alpha\beta$ chains. The antigen binding site of the TCR is encoded by the recombined VDJ segments of the β, δ and VJ of the α, γ TCR genes. The regions of the TCR molecule that form the complementary surface with the antigen are termed *complementary determining regions*, or CDRs. Thus, the three CDRs of TCR, CDR1, CDR2, and CDR3, form the antigen binding site. CDR3 is in the center, displays most diversity, and directly interacts with the antigens, while CDR1 and CDR2 are in the periphery and interact with the α helices of the MHC molecules (see page 27).

As we discussed in Chap. 5, the diversity of the TCR as with immunoglobulins is generated by gene rearrangement. For the TCR α and γ chains, the CDRs are the final products of VJ rearrangement, and for TCR β and δ, the CDRs are generated by the recombination of the VDJ segments. In the gene rearrangement process, the additions of nucleotides at each junction of each segment further increase TCR diversity and expand the TCR repertoire. The addition of nucleotides is catalyzed by the enzyme *terminal deoxynucleotidyltransferase (TdT)* and does not require DNA template. Thus, these nucleotides are termed *N-region nucleotides (Non-template nucleotides)*. Once rearranged, the coding sequence of each TCR remains unchanged and does not display somatic hypermutation as with B cell-derived immunoglobulins.

At the cell surface level of T cells, TCRs are expressed as heterodimers of either $\alpha\beta$ or $\gamma\delta$. No other combinations or single chain TCR has ever been found expressed by T cells. All the four TCR chains are integral cell membrane molecules displaying an extracellular domain, a transmembrane domain, and a short cytoplasmic tail. The extracellular domains consist of variable, constant, and hinge regions. The three CDRs reside within the variable region. The CDR3 displays the highest diversity generated by the joining of D and J segments and the addition of N-region nucleotides to each junction. In contrast, the CDR1 and CDR2 are encoded by the $V\alpha$ and $V\beta$ genes. The CDR3 forms the center of the antigen binding site, while the CDR1 and CDR2 form the periphery of the antigen binding site and display relatively less diversity. When a TCR engages antigen-MHC complexes on an APC, the CDR3 binds directly to the antigenic

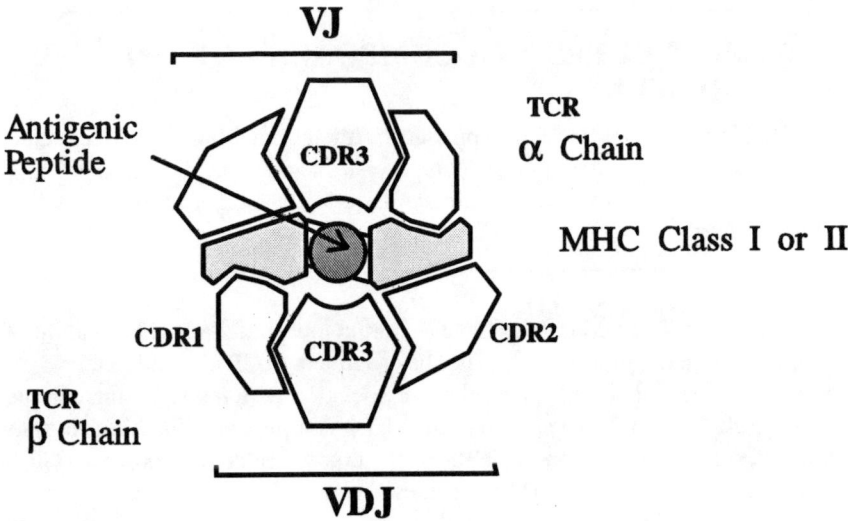

Figure 8-1
The outline structure showing the horizontal cross section of the TCR CDR1, CDR2 and
CDR3 when the TCR binds to an antigenic peptide in the groove of MHC I or MHC II.
The CDR3 which displays most diversity binds to the antigenic peptide, while the CDR1
and CDR2 bind to the α helices of the two outer MHC domains.

peptide, and the CDR1 and CDR2 contact the α helices of the two outer MHC
domains (Fig. 8-1). It has been suggested that the limited numbers of the V gene
segments generate diversity needed for recognition of MHC molecules and the
great diversity generated at the junctional regions, ensuring recognition of most
antigenic peptides.

SUPERANTIGENS

Superantigens are a unique class of antigen from bacteria and viruses that
have the ability to bind to the TCR-MHC complex in a less stringent fashion and to activate large numbers of T cells, resulting in various severe ill-
nesses such as food poisoning and toxic shock syndrome.

Although most antigenic peptides are presented to the TCR by inserting
between two helices of the MHC molecules, the superantigens bind to the lateral
surfaces of either MHC I or MHC II. Furthermore, they bind directly to the portion of the TCR encoded by the Vβ genes that are not part of the antigen binding
sites (CDR3). It is important to note that binding of superantigen to TCR $\alpha\beta$ is
independent of the α chain and the DJ segments of the Vβ chains, the segment
that encodes the CDR3.

CD3 MOLECULES AS A COMPONENT OF THE TCR COMPLEX

The TCR molecules are not expressed by themselves but are associated with the signal-transducing CD3 complexes. The CD3 has five chains that combine to form four distinct dimers: $\gamma\epsilon$, $\delta\epsilon$, and $\zeta\eta$ heterodimers and $\zeta\zeta$ homodimers.

The four TCR glycoproteins have a short cytoplasmic tail with no ability to transduce an activation signal. The heterodimers TCR$\alpha\beta$ and TCR$\gamma\delta$ are expressed on the cell surface of T cells in association with the signaling complex CD3 (Figs. 8-2 and 8-3). Expression of the CD3 complex also functions in stabilizing cell surface expression of TCR; T cells do not effectively express TCR on the cell surface without the CD3 molecules.

The five CD3 chains and TCR α, β, δ, and γ are members of the *immunoglobulin superfamily*. All members of the TCR have two immunoglobulin-like extracellular domains (see Chap. 3). In contrast, the CD3 γ, δ, and ϵ chains have only one extracellular domain. The TCR extracellular domains are followed by a transmembrane and a short cytoplasmic tail. One unique feature of the transmembrane domain of the TCR is the presence of positively charged amino acids that bind to the negatively charged transmembrane domains of the CD3 γ, δ, and ϵ chains and stabilize the TCR-CD3 complex (Appendix 1).

The CD3ζ and η chains are products of the same genes and are generated by alternate splicing, resulting in different carboxyl termini. The CD3 ζ and η chains are not members of the immunoglobulin superfamily and have only a short extracellular domain. In 80 to 90% of TCR-CD3 complexes, the ζ chains are present as $\zeta\zeta$ homodimers; the $\zeta\eta$ heterodimers are only found on the remaining 10 to 20% of the T cells.

SIGNAL-TRANSDUCING COMPONENTS OF THE CD3-TCR COMPLEX

Two receptor-associated protein-tyrosine kinases have been found associated with the TCR-CD3 complex. Fyn has been found associated with the CD3ϵ, and a protein of 70 kD termed ζ-*associated protein-70* (*ZAP-70*) bound to the $\zeta\zeta$ homodimers. When activated, these protein-tyrosine kinases phosphorylate a series of target molecules including CD3 molecules as well as ZAP-70.

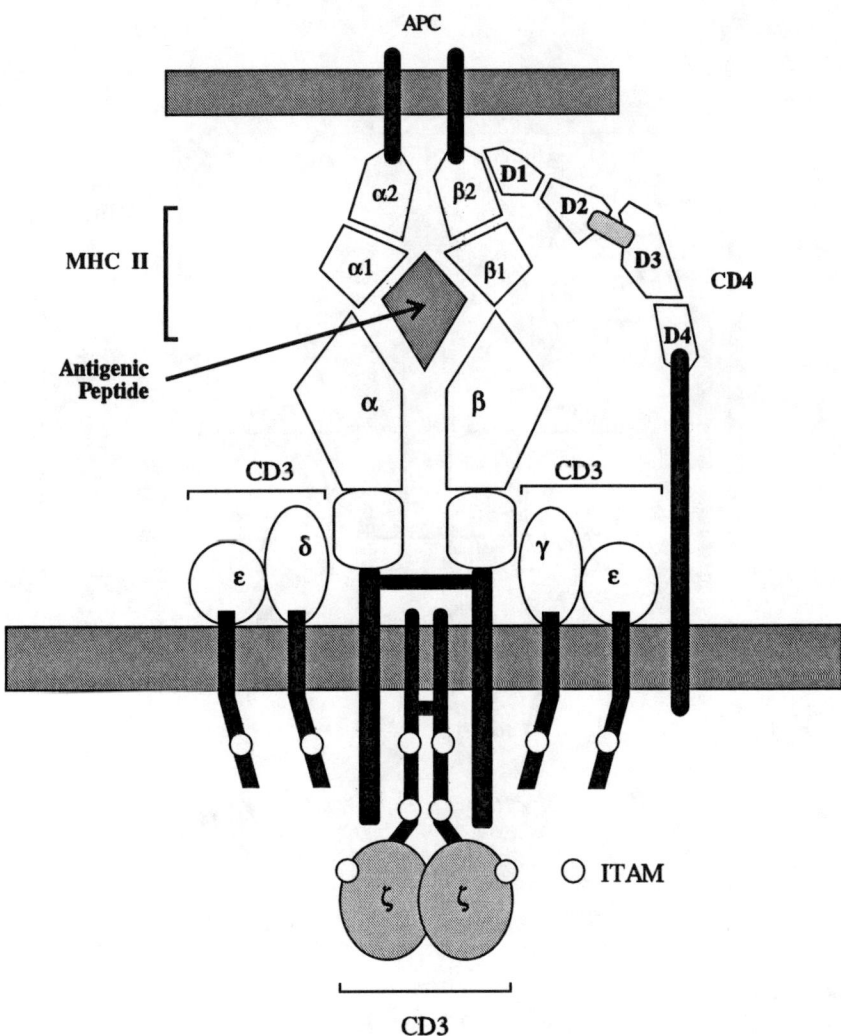

Figure 8-2

Structure of the CD4 co-receptor-CD3-TCR complex expressed on the cell surface of the CD4 positive T cells. The CD4 molecule with four immunoglobulin-like domains (D1-D4) binds simultaneously to the β2 domain of the MCH II when TCR engages an antigenic peptide presented by antigen presenting cells (APC). The CD3 cytoplasmic tails of ε, δ, γ, and ξ display ITAM domains; there is more ITAM in the ξ chain than in the other CD3 chains.

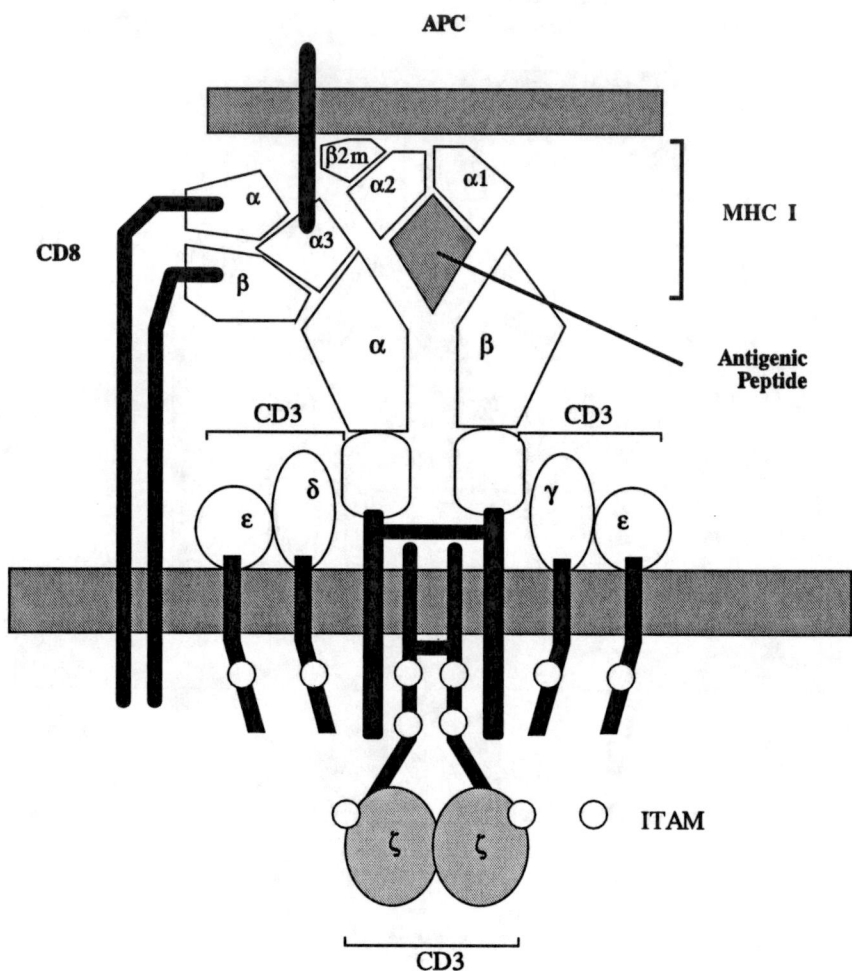

Figure 8-3
Structure of the CD8 co-receptor-CD3-TCR complex expressed on the cell surface of the CD8 positive T cells. Both of the CD8 α, β chains bind to the α3 domain of the MHC I molecules when TCR engages an antigenic peptide presented by APC.

     All five chains of the CD3 molecules contain a conserved region in the cytoplasmic tail that functions in signal transduction. The conserved domain is termed the *immune receptor tyrosine-based activation motif* (*ITAM*) and contains a pair of tyrosine and leucine residues. The tyrosine residues are substrates for the protein-tyrosine kinases during activation of T cells. The CD3 γ, δ, ϵ chains have only one ITAM in their cytoplasmic tail, while the ζ and η have three copies of ITAM. When phosphorylated, these regions lead to the recruitment of more ZAP-70 to the TCR-CD3 complex and also to activation of ZAP-70.

CD4 AND CD8 CO-RECEPTORS

Although the TCR-CD3 is directly responsible for binding to the antigen-MHC complex and delivering signals into the cells, optimal binding and activation of T cells requires co-receptors and accessory cell surface molecules. CD4 and CD8 are important co-receptors for TCR binding to MHC II and MHC I, respectively, as well as activation of T cells. Both CD4 and CD8 are associated with the protein-tyrosine kinase lck.

Through the process of positive selection (see Chap. 5), T cells matured in the thymus are selected according to the ability of their TCR to bind to MHC I and II molecules. The ability to bind MHC I or II is dictated by the CD8 and CD4, respectively. Thus, CD4 binds to the invariable domain of the MHC II, while CD8 binds to the invariable domain of the MHC I (see Figs. 8-2 and 8-3). For this reason, the CD4 and CD8 molecules are named the *TCR co-receptors*.

Both CD4 and CD8 are also members of the immunoglobulin superfamily. The CD4 molecule contains four immunoglobulin-like domains (D1 to D4); the first two domains are separated from D3 and D4 by a hinge region. The CD4 is expressed as a single chain membrane protein (see Fig. 8-2). In contrast, CD8 is expressed as $\alpha\beta$ heterodimers or as $\alpha\alpha$ homodimers. Furthermore, the extracellular portion of the CD8 molecules has only one immunoglobulin-like domain (see Fig. 8-3). The cytoplasmic tails of both CD4 and CD8 are associated with lck.

When TCR-CD3 of a $CD4^+$ T cell engages MHC II molecules on APC, the D1 domain of the CD4 molecules simultaneously binds to the $\beta2$ domain of the MHC II (see Fig. 8-2). Similarly, the $\alpha\beta$ portion of the CD8 molecules binds to the MHC I $\alpha3$ domain when $CD8^+$ T cells recognize antigen presented by APC (see Fig. 8-3). Both the binding of CD4 to MHC I and CD8 to MHC I stabilizes T cell-APC cognate interaction and facilitates activation of T cells. The activation of T cells is mediated by a receptor-associated protein-tyrosine kinase, lck, that is associated with the cytoplasmic tails of CD4 and CD8 molecules.

In addition to the CD4 and CD8 co-receptors, there are other accessory molecules expressed on T cells and APC that participate in the activation of T cells. The accessory molecules function as ligand-receptor pairs that participate in both cell-cell adhesion and signal transduction. A list of well documented accessory molecules is provided in Table 8-1.

TABLE 8-1
T CELL ACCESSORY MOLECULES

T CELLS	APC
CD2	LFA-3 (CD58)
LFA-1 (CD11a/CD18)	ICAM-1 (CD54)
CD28	B7.1 (CD80)
CTLA-4	B7.2 (CD86)
CD5	CD72
CD45	CD22

T CELL ACTIVATION

To carry out effector functions such as CD4 T cell helper activity or CD8 cytotoxic activity, T cells need to be activated. T cell activation is initiated by aggregation of TCR-CD3 complexes caused by antigen binding. This aggregation activates a cell surface protein phosphatase (CD45), a series of receptor-associated protein-tyrosine kinases, and protein kinase C (PKC). These intracellular events subsequently activate a series of transcription factors that translocate to the nucleus and initiate transcription of important cytokines and cytokine receptors.

Mature T cells, when they leave the thymus, remain inactive in the G_0 phase of the cell cycle. These T cells that have not yet encountered any foreign antigens are *naive T cells*. The naive T cells, when they recognize an antigen-MHC complex on an appropriate APC, will be activated, initiating a primary response. As a consequence of the primary response, effector or activated T cells and memory T cells are generated. Activated T cells have a short life and will die by apoptosis 2 to 3 days after the primary response. On the contrary, memory cells have a longer life span (months to years) and respond vigorously with the same antigen in the subsequent antigenic challenging, the secondary response (see Chap. 9).

When sufficient numbers of TCR-CD3 molecules engage with antigen-MHC complexes, aggregation of TCR-CD3 complexes at the cell surface level occurs and results in the recruitment of additional co-receptors, like CD4 or CD8, and accessory molecule CD45 to the receptor complexes. It was estimated that aggregation of approximately 100 TCR-CD3 molecules is sufficient to initiate T cell activation.

Within the close proximity of the receptor aggregate, CD45, which functions as a protein phosphatase, activates the protein-tyrosine kinases lck and fyn. The targets of the two protein-tyrosine kinases are the ITAM domains presented in the CD3 γ, δ, ϵ, and γ chains. When ζ chains are phosphorylated, they recruit and activate ZAP-70, itself also a protein-tyrosine kinase. The next enzyme activated by ZAP-70 is the phospholipase Cγ-1 (PLC-γ1). PLC-γ generates two active molecules from the phosphatidylinositol biphosphate (PIP2): inositol triphosphate (IP3) and diacylglycerol (DAG). DAG in turn activates PKC, while IP3 induces release of Ca^{2+} from the endoplasmic reticulum, raising the intracellular levels of Ca^{2+}. The last cytoplasmic event in this cascade reaction is the activation of two important transcription factors, the *NF-κB* (nuclear factor that binds the κ light chain regulatory region) and NF-AT (nuclear factor of activated T cells). Activation of NF-κB is dependent on PKC, while NF-AT activation is dependent on calcineurin, a calmodulin-dependent phosphatase. The two most potent inhibitors of calcineurin are *cyclosporin-A* and *FK-506*. The two drugs can effectively inhibit T cell activation and are widely used as immunosuppressive drugs. Activated transcription factors then translocate to the nucleus.

The final phase of T cell activation takes place in the nucleus, where activated transcription factors bind to regulator regions of various cytokines and cytokine receptors and initiate new transcription. One of the most important cytokine and cytokine receptor is IL2 and IL2 receptor that function to maintain survival of the activated T cells. A list of other cytokines produced by activated T cells are shown in Table 8-2.

TABLE 8-2
**CYTOKINES PRODUCED BY AND RECEPTOR FOUND
ON ACTIVATED T CELLS**

IL2	IL2 receptor (CD25)
IL3	IL4
IL5	IL6
IFN-γ	TNF-α

HUMORAL IMMUNITY

•

• • • • • • • • • • • •

HUMORAL IMMUNITY

Humoral immunity involves the production by an immunized donor of soluble proteins called antibodies that can be transferred in the donor serum to an unimmunized recipient to confer immediate specific immunity within the recipient. This is in contrast to cellular immunity, which involves the transfer of whole cells from the donor to confer immunity in the recipient.

The antibodies produced against an antigen during a humoral immune response in an immunized donor can provide immediate protection to an unimmunized recipient against a specific antigen. For example, a person bitten by a snake can receive immediate protection from the serum of a donor that had previously mounted a humoral immune response against the snake bite venom. The advantage to this passive transfer of immunity to the snake bite victim is that the victim himself does not have to wait the 5 to 6 days required for optimal antibody production to occur against this specific antigen. However, for most antigens entering the body, the initial production of antibody does occur within the host. Therefore, an understanding of how antibody production occurs is essential to our understanding of one basic protective mechanism that we have for neutralizing antigens.

MECHANISMS BY WHICH ANTIBODIES PROVIDE IMMUNITY

Neutralization of antigen
Fc receptor-mediated phagocytosis
Complement-mediated lysis

There are three primary mechanisms by which antibodies confer immunity. First, antibodies can bind to soluble or cell-associated antigens to prevent their inducing any detrimental effects. For example, the HIV expresses a number of antigens that stimulate the production of specific antibodies. The antibodies produced are then able to bind to the cell surface antigens, present on an intact virus, that initially stimulated their production. Since some of these HIV-associated antigens are important for the virus to gain entry into a host CD4+ T cell, the binding of a specific antibody to these antigens will neutralize the ability of the virus to enter a T cell.

OPSONIZATION

Opsonization is the process of coating an antigen with specific antibody to promote phagocytosis of the antigen.

Second, antibodies can bind to soluble and cell-associated antigens and, subsequently, bind to phagocytic cells via the Fc portion of the antibody to the Fc receptor expressed on phagocytic cells. In this manner, the antibody coating the antigen delivers the antigen to the phagocyte and thereby enhances both the phagocytosis and the ultimate destruction of the antigen by these cells. Third, antibodies can bind to cell-associated antigens and, subsequently, activate complement proteins that form pores in the cell to destroy the cell through lysis. The process of coating an antigen with specific antibody to promote phagocytosis is known as *opsonization*.

PRIMARY AND SECONDARY ANTIBODY RESPONSES

PRIMARY	SECONDARY
Response to first antigen exposure	Response to second antigen exposure
Lag time in response	Immediate response
IgM	IgG
Low affinity antibody	High affinity antibody

Antigen exposure for the first time induces an antibody response that can be measured in the serum after a lag period of about 6 to 12 days (Fig. 9-1). The antibody isotype produced during a primary response is mostly IgM, the level of antibody produced decreases shortly after peak levels have been obtained, and the generation of memory B cells occurs. In contrast, exposure to the same antigen a second time induces an antibody response that can be measured in the serum within a few days of antigen exposure. The antibody isotype produced is primarily IgG, the level of antibody in the serum persists from weeks to months after antigen exposure, and the affinity of the antibody for antigen is greatly increased.

The process of antibody formation is a complex and intricate phenomenon. The B cell is the cell ultimately responsible for making antibody. However, the production of antibody by B cells can occur in either a T cell-independent or a T cell-dependent manner, depending on the nature of the antigen eliciting the response. The classification of these antigens depends on whether or not an antibody response can be generated in a thymus-deficient host. Since the thymus is responsible for generating all the mature T cells that are used to elicit immune responses in the body, an antigen that generates an antibody response in a host lacking a thymus is classified as a T cell-independent antigen, as opposed to an antigen that is T cell-dependent and requires the presence of a thymus to generate an antibody response.

T CELL-INDEPENDENT AND -DEPENDENT ANTIGENS

T cell-independent antigens are antigens that activate B cells in a polyclonal manner in the absence of CD4+ T-helper cells. *T-cell dependent antigens* are antigens that activate B cells only in the presence of CD4+ T-helper cells.

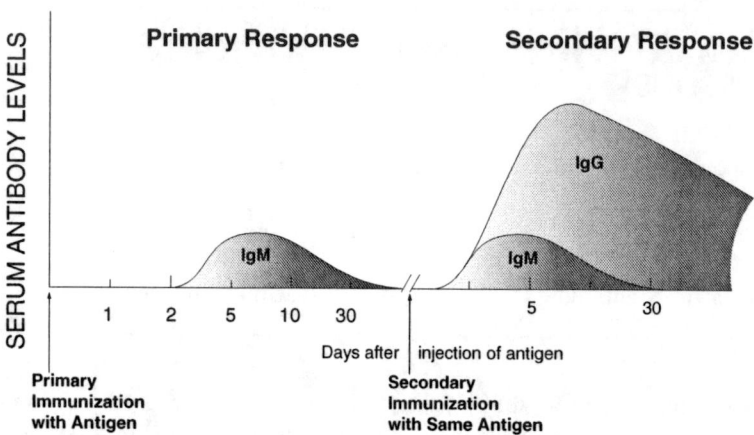

Figure 9-1
Primary and secondary antibody responses

T cell-independent antigens activate B cells in a *polyclonal* manner; i.e., they activate many different B cells regardless of their epitope specificity and do not necessarily activate B cells through interaction with the immunoglobulin receptor. In this manner, T cell-independent antigens induce B cells to produce antibodies that will bind to many different antigenic determinants, even those to which the B cell was not exposed. T cell-independent antigens include the lipopolysaccharides of Gram-negative bacteria and other antigens in which an immunodominant epitope is repeated many times, such as polymeric proteins. T cell-independent antigens induce primarily IgM production and do not induce B cell memory.

In contrast, a B cell response to low concentrations of T cell-dependent antigens requires the presence of CD4+ T-helper cells. In this manner, either a hapten or a particular epitope of a soluble protein antigen is recognized by the antigen binding site of the immunoglobulin molecule on the cell surface of a B cell, and, therefore, B cells are selected in an antigen-specific manner. However, this selected B cell cannot make antibody until a T cell recognizes a unique epitope of either the soluble protein antigen or the carrier protein attached to the hapten, both of which must first undergo extensive degradation. This process of degradation occurs only after antigens enter the cell through B cell-mediated endocytosis. Once inside the B cell, the antigen is processed and reexpressed on the surface of the B cell in association with gene products of the MHC class II as has been described in detail in Chap. 7. The selective recognition of different epitopes on the same immunogen by T and B lymphocytes forces these two different lymphocytes to physically interact with each other to activate each other to induce *clonal expansion*; i.e., single antigen-specific T and B cells will proliferate to produce clones of themselves, all of which produce the same type of cytokine and antibody. T cell-dependent antigens induce both primary and memory B cell antibody responses leading to the production of IgM, IgG, IgA, and IgE antibodies. More importantly, these different classes of antibodies bind only to the specific antigen that originally bound to the immunoglobulin molecule expressed on the cell surface of the antibody-producing B cell.

THEORIES OF HOW ANTIGEN-SPECIFIC ANTIBODIES ARE MADE

These previous theories have been disproved.

Selective theory: multiple immunoglobulin specificities expressed by one B cell.

Instructive theory: antigen molds the specificity of the immunoglobulin molecule.

These current theories are accepted.

Clonal selection theory: immunoglobulin diversity is generated before antigen enters the system.

Network theory: involves a process of idiotype-anti-idiotype antibody interactions.

Before discussing the detailed mechanism by which B cells become activated to produce antigen-specific antibody against a T cell-dependent antigen, the different theories that have been proposed to be responsible for antibody formation must be fully understood. The *selective theory* proposed that an antigen combined with one out of several molecules on the surface of immune cells stimulates the generation and release of that one particular molecule more than others. This theory became invalid when it was realized that each cell would be required to express a vast number of different molecules to recognize a vast number of structurally different natural and synthetic antigens. In contrast, the *instructive theory* proposed that antigen acted as a template for instructing a nonspecific antibody on the cell surface to fold itself around the antigen to make a specific antibody against that antigen. This theory was challenged when it was determined that antibody specificity lies in the primary amino acid sequence of the antibody protein molecule.

The most accepted theory to date is known as the *clonal selection theory*. This theory proposes that antigen receptor diversity is generated before antigen enters the system and that the role of antigen is to selectively stimulate specific receptors on a specific clone of cells to induce these cells to proliferate and produce specific antibody against the antigen. This theory implies that all secreted antibody produced by cells from the expanded clone will have antigen-combining sites identical to the antibody receptors on the surface of the original clone. Thus, all of the antibody produced against a single antigen is the result of the selection, activation, and expansion of cells expressing a restricted antigen receptor specificity.

Clonal selection can also be induced by a mechanism that does not involve external antigen but instead involves a process of idiotype-anti-idiotype antibody interactions. This mechanism of antibody production is known as the *network theory*. This theory proposes that each immunoglobulin molecule expresses its own unique set of determinants within the variable domain, each of which is called an *idiotope*. Collectively, all of the individual idiotopes make up the antibody idiotype. The idiotype is recognized as foreign by immunoglobulin molecules expressed on other cells, and these antibodies are known as anti-idiotypic antibody molecules. The idiotopes of the anti-idiotype antibodies are, in turn, recognized by other immunoglobulin molecules expressed on other cells; thus, a network of interacting cells is established. In this manner, idiotype-anti-idiotype interaction limits the clonal expansion of B cells and, thus, keeps these cells in a state of equilibrium. Since the idiotope mimics the image of an external foreign antigen, the idiotype-anti-idiotype interaction can be broken by the entry of external antigen into the system. The specific antigen breaks the state of equilibrium established by the idiotype-anti-idiotype interactions and induces a specific set of B cells to clonally expand.

ANTIGEN-SPECIFIC T CELL-DEPENDENT ANTIBODY FORMATION

This is the production of antibody against a specific antigen by a specific B cell and only in the presence of T cells that recognize a processed form of the same antigen.

The clonal selection theory laid the foundation for studies establishing that B cells express immunoglobulin molecules that bind antigens and then proceed through a sequence of activation, proliferation, and differentiation events that culminate in the production of antibodies that neutralize and/or eliminate the antigens that initially triggered their activation. However, the B cell requires "help" to proceed through this sequence of activation events. CD4+ T cells provide this help. Initially, as shown in Fig. 9-2, the B cell functions *independently* of CD4+ T cells to bind, endocytose, and process antigen into small fragments. These small antigenic fragments are then reexpressed on the B cell surface in association with MHC class II. After these events, B cell function is *dependent* on the presence of CD4+ T cells. The CD4+ T cell receptor recognizes the processed antigen-MHC complex on the B cell surface and tightly interacts with the B cell.

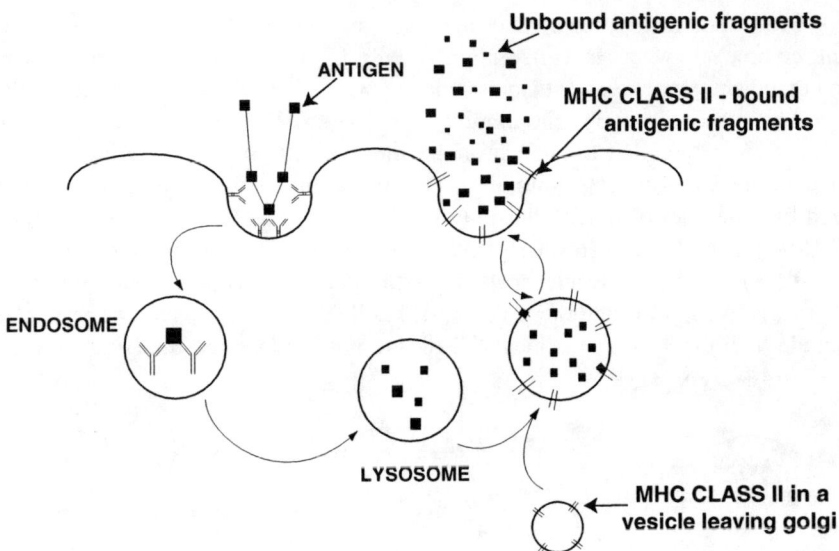

Figure 9-2
Antigen processing by a B cell.

The intimate cell-cell interaction that occurs allows for the transduction of signals across the membrane of both the CD4+ T cell and B cell to induce lymphokine release by the CD4+ T cell and a state of lymphokine responsiveness in the B cell. In this manner, only antigen-specific B cells become activated to respond to the cytokines that are released in their immediate environment. At this point, the B cells respond to the T cell-derived cytokines by clonally expanding and, days later, secreting antigen-specific antibody.

T CELL-B CELL INTERACTION MOLECULES THAT ARE IMPORTANT FOR T CELL-DEPENDENT ANTIBODY PRODUCTION

T CELL	*B CELL*
T Cell Receptor/CD4	Antigen/MHC Class II
CD2	CD58 (LFA-3)
CD54 (ICAM-1)	CD11/CD18 (LFA-1 α/β)
CD11/CD18 (LFA-1 α/β)	CD54 (ICAM-1)
CD28	CD80 (B7.1)/CD86 (B7.2)
CD40L	CD40

More specifically, the contact-mediated signals to activate the T cell and B cell commence when B cells interact with CD4+ T cells as they present processed antigenic fragments in association with MHC class II molecules to the T cell receptor (Fig. 9-3). The binding of CD4 to MHC class II and of CD2 to CD58 (formerly called LFA-3) promote the initiation of the signaling process through the T cell receptor complex. This initial interaction is further strengthened by a number of other adhesion molecules, such as CD54 (formerly called ICAM-1) and CD11/18 (formerly called LFA-1 α/β) present on the cell surface of both cells. Other molecules, called co-stimulatory molecules, are required for optimal activation of both the T cell and B cell. These co-stimulatory molecules include both the T cell-associated CD28 that is stimulated by the B cell-associ-

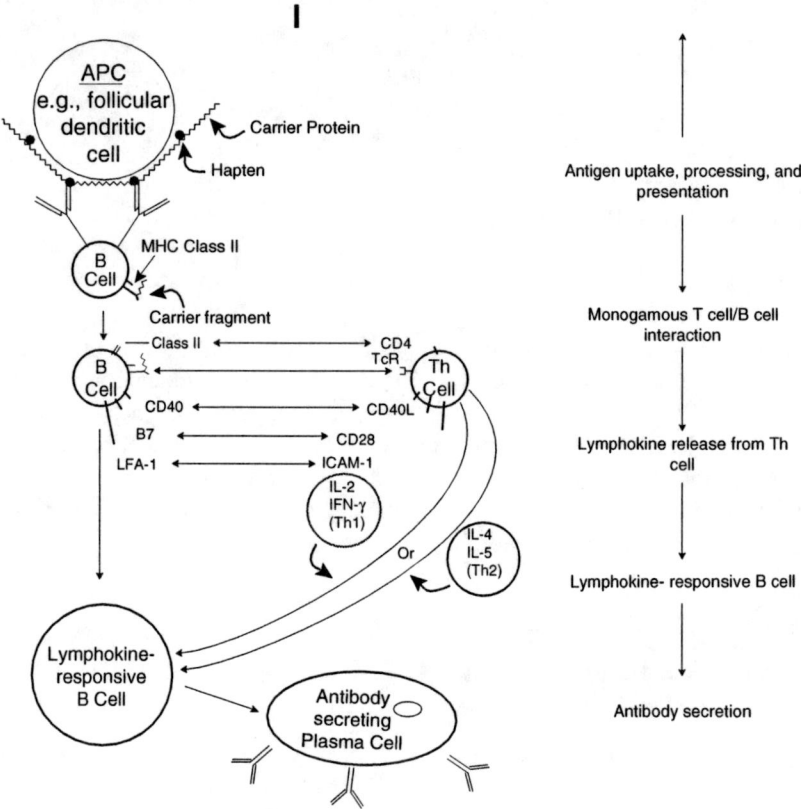

Figure 9-3
Interaction between APC, B cell, and Th cell in generating an antibody-secreting plasma cell.

ated CD80 (formerly called B7.1) or CD86 (formerly called B7.2) and the B cell-associated CD40 molecule that is stimulated by the T cell-associated CD40L molecule. Interestingly, it is the CD28-CD86 co-stimulatory signal that appears to be responsible for activation of the T cell to express the CD40L molecule that is critical to B cell activation via stimulation of the CD40 molecule. The lack of CD40L expression on immune cells leads to the development of a disease in humans known as X-linked hyper-IgM syndrome. As part of the clinical symptoms associated with this syndrome, the host is unable to generate high affinity IgG antibodies to combat extracellular bacteria and, thus, succumbs to severe bacterial infections. Diseases such as this one have helped us to understand the physiological significance of the CD40L-CD40 interaction between a T cell and B cell that was initially characterized in a test tube.

CYTOKINE PROFILES AND ANTIBODY ISOTYPE PRODUCTION

Th1 cell → IL-2 and IFN-γ → IgM and IgG2a

Th2 cell → IL-4, IL-5, IL-6, IL-10 → IgM and IgG4 (IgG1 in the mouse)

Moreover, CD4+ T-helper (Th) cells not only activate the B cell during cell-cell interaction, but they also provide the cytokines necessary for B cell growth and differentiation into antibody-secreting cells. Two CD4+ Th cell subsets have been identified and are characterized by the cytokines they secrete. Th1 cells secrete interleukin (IL)-2 and interferon (IFN)-γ, while Th2 cells secrete IL-4, IL-5, IL-6, and IL-10. Both CD4+ T cell subsets provide help for B cell IgM production, albeit to different degrees, while their distinctive cytokines influence the production of particular antibody isotypes. For example, *in vivo*, mice that produce high amounts of IFN-γ and little IL-4 produce large amounts of IgG_{2a}, while mice that produce high amounts of IL-4 and little IFN-γ produce large amounts of IgG_1. *In vitro*, IFN-γ-producing Th1 cells induce B cells to produce IgG_{2a}, while IL-4-producing Th2 cells induce B cells to produce IgG_1. However, maximal T cell-dependent antibody production is induced by a combination of cytokines released from both CD4+ T cell subsets.

The important point to remember is that as a result of the above-described scenario, a specific B cell will be activated to produce antibody only against the antigen that bound to the B cell immunoglobulin molecule initially. It is also important to note that the T cell and B cell become activated as a consequence of recognizing the same antigen, albeit as a consequence of recognizing different epitopes on that same antigen.

INFLAMMATION

·

- **The Inflammatory Process**
- **Acute Inflammation**
- **Chemotaxis**
- **Adhesion Molecules**
- **Inflammatory Mediators**
- **Chronic Inflammation**

THE INFLAMMATORY PROCESS

The inflammatory process is the body's response to injury, triggered by invasion of bacteria or other infectious agents.

The inflammatory reaction occurs independent of the immune system after physical injury. It is characterized by 1) increased blood flow to the affected area, to dilute potentially toxic agents, 2) increased capillary permeability, to facilitate transmission of larger molecules across the endothelium, and 3) the migration of leukocytes (primarily neutrophils and to a lesser extent macrophages) out of the circulatory system between endothelial cells by *diapedesis* into the surrounding tissue (Fig. 10-1). These processes are initiated within minutes (Fig. 10-2) but the consequences can linger for weeks to months. The goal of the leukocytes is to remove debris and restore normal tissue structure and function. A subset of these cells are capable of phagocytosis, and they perform this function by internalizing and digesting necrotic tissue as well as foreign material. The duration and magnitude of the inflammatory response dictates the ultimate outcome. If the tissue is more severely damaged and the inflammatory response is prolonged, then it will be more difficult to restore normal tissue architecture.

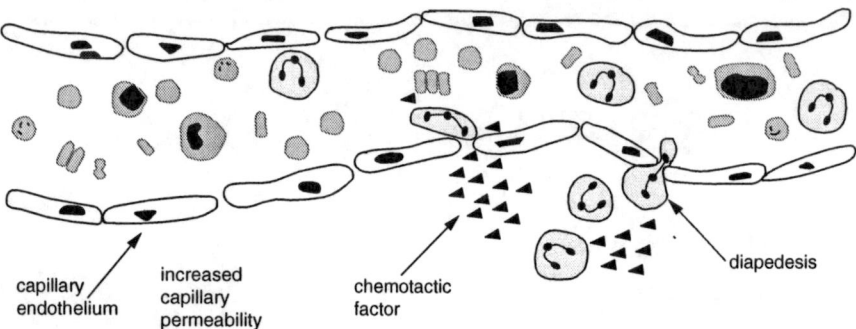

Figure 10-1
Acute inflammatory response.

ACUTE INFLAMMATION

Acute inflammation is the early phase of the inflammatory process, characterized by

Rubor (redness)
Calor (heat)
Tumor (swelling, edema)
Dolor (pain)

Leukocytes (see Chap. 2), which normally constitute 1% of the circulating cells, with the remaining being primarily RBCs, are active in the repair process that follows tissue injury and in fighting infection. The first cell type to appear at an inflammatory site is the *neutrophil*, a subset of polymorphonuclear leukocytes (PMNs) or "polys" (Table 10-1). At sites of inflammation, neutrophils adhere to the walls of postcapillary venules and diapedese between the endothelial cells into the connective tissue matrix below. Once at their target site, neutrophils exert their effects by releasing the contents of their cytoplasmic granules, which contain hydrolytic enzymes and reactive oxygen metabolites. In addition, neutrophils are avid phagocytic cells especially effective against bacteria. The contents of

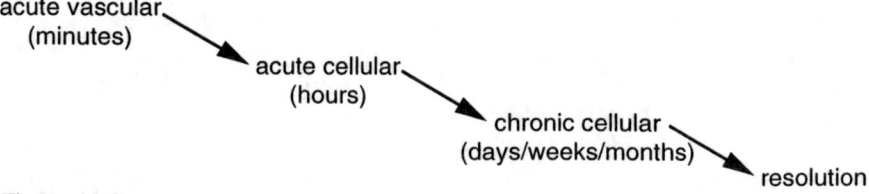

Figure 10-2
Timing of the cascade of inflammatory events.

TABLE 10-1
CHARACTERISTICS OF INFLAMMATORY CELLS

CELL TYPE	DIAMETER	FREQUENCY IN BLOOD %	NUCLEAR MORPHOLOGY	GRANULES
Neutrophil	9–12 μm	60–70	Multilobed	Neutral staining
Mast cells	10–30 μm		Large, round, centrally located	Large metachromatic staining
Eosinophils	10–14 μm	2–4	Bi/multilobed	Red-Orange staining
Basophils	8–10 μm	0.5–1	Bilobed or U-shaped	Large metachromatic or basophilic
Monocytes	12–15 μm	3–8	Oval or kidney bean-shaped	None
Lymphocytes	8–10 μm	20–35	Dense, round, eccentrically located	None

their phagocytic vacuoles fuse with lysosomes containing hydrolytic enzymes to digest the contents.

Mast cells, located in perivascular connective tissue throughout the body, are most commonly known for their role in *Type I hypersensitivity reactions* or *immediate hypersensitivity* (Chap. 12). Since they have high affinity cell surface receptors for the Fc portion of the immunoglobulin molecules, mast cells are capable of fixation of IgE and antigen (Fig. 10-3). This causes mast cells to degranulate, thus releasing their chemical mediators.

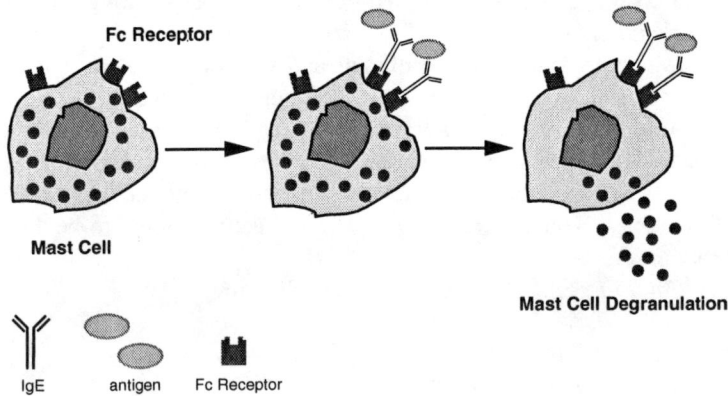

Figure 10-3
Mast cell degranulation.

Functions triggered by mast cell activation include the following.

Histamine: increase in the blood flow and capillary permeability
Heparin: decrease in blood coagulability
Slow releasing factors of anaphylaxis (SRS-A):   increase in muscle tone
Prostaglandins: pain, contraction of smooth muscle cells
Chemotactic factors: recruitment of neutrophil and eosinophil

Eosinophils are involved in *allergic responses* (Chap. 12) and aid in the resistance to *parasitic infection* (Chap. 15). They are commonly found in the connective tissue of the digestive and respiratory systems, as well as in the circulation during allergic responses (asthma and hay fever) and following parasitic infection. In addition to their role in acute inflammatory processes, eosinophils are also present in chronic inflammation, although the numbers of cells may be quite low. They do not directly phagocytose bacteria or other particulate antigens directly, but they do take up antigen-antibody complexes. Furthermore, they release pharmacologically active mediators that increase vascular permeability, including serotonin and prostaglandins. Finally, eosinophils play a critical role in the response to parasitic infection. Major basic protein, which is contained in the granules of eosinophils, is released upon degranulation. The protein coats the cell surface of the parasites and facilitates antibody-dependent killing of the organisms. It also acts on mast cells to cause their degeneration.

Basophils resemble the connective tissue mast cell in both structure and function, yet they arise from different lineages. Both are involved in increasing the permeability of the vascular system during inflammation and bind immunoglobulin, primarily IgE. Degranulation occurs in allergic reactions following the binding of antigen-bound immunoglobulin to the cell surface. The granules contain agents that are chemotactic for leukocytes, as well as histamine, which causes vasodilation and promotes the migration of those cells from the circulatory system to the connective tissue. This can cause local swelling and in extreme cases *anaphylactic shock*.

In addition to leukocytes, epithelial and connective tissue cells, such as fibroblasts, once thought of as passive bystanders in inflammatory events, are now known to play critical roles in both acute and chronic inflammation. These roles include the expression of cell surface adhesion molecules (which mediate the adherence between the leukocytes and the endothelial cells) and the production of cytokines, which recruit leukocytes and activate them to better perform their functions.

The *Capillary Endothelium* acts as the following.

A selectively permeable barrier
A synthetic and metabolic system
A nonthrombogenic container for blood

Capillary *endothelial cells*, a subclass of epithelial cells that surround the lumen of blood vessels, provide the barrier between the connective tissue and the vascular system. Under abnormal conditions, such as inflammation, capillary and post capillary venular permeability is greatly increased. This is achieved by altering the state of the junctional complexes between adjacent endothelial cells, thus allowing leukocytes to leave the blood stream by passing between endothelial cells and entering the underlying tissue by a process called *diapedesis* (see Fig. 10-1). The local release of mediators, including histamine and bradykinin, facilitates diapedesis by increasing the permeability across the endothelial cell layer.

Upon activation, capillary endothelial cells can produce cell adhesion molecules and a variety of cytokines that allow for the margination of leukocytes prior to their migration from the blood vessel to the site of inflammation.

CHEMOTAXIS

Chemotaxis is the directed migration along a concentration gradient, as opposed to chemokinesis or cytokinesis, which involve random cell movement.

A key element in the inflammatory process is *chemotaxis*. Cells are diverted from the vascular system to sites of tissue damage by chemotactic factors, which are generated at the site of inflammation and diffuse laterally. By design they are small molecules with short half-lives to readily permit their diffusion and the termination of their effects.

The first such factor to be described was *C5a*, a reactive glycopeptide produced in both the classical and alternative pathways of the complement cascade (see Chap. 14). C5a is chemotactic for neutrophils and macrophages at nanomolar concentrations. Other chemotactic mediators include formyl peptides (f-Met-Leu-Phe), leukotriene B_4, thrombin, transforming growth factor β (TGFβ), interleukin-8 (IL-8), monocyte chemotactic peptide (MCP-1), and platelet-activating factor (PAF) and the connective tissue proteins, fibronectin, collagen, laminin, and fragments of elastin. Thus, both blood-borne agents and components of disrupted basement membranes can serve to attract cells to the extravascular space.

ADHESION MOLECULES

Adhesion molecules are cell surface molecules that are present on both leukocytes and endothelial cells and are thought to mediate adhesive interactions between those cell populations.

In order for cells to migrate to and through endothelial cell monolayers, adhesion must take place. While endothelial cells attach to one another by means of junctional complexes, leukocytes do not. They utilize a set of cell surface molecules called *cell adhesion molecules* or *CAMs*. In response to chemotactic signals, selectins on the surface of circulating leukocytes interact with selectins on the luminal surface of endothelial cells. This loose association is called *tethering*. The leukocytes then roll along the endothelial cell surface and either fall off of the cell due to the shear force of blood flow or firmly adhere to the endothelial cell. Firm adhesion is mediated by integrins. This is then followed by *emigration* of leukocytes between the endothelial cells by *diapedesis*. Cytokines and bacterial products up-regulate the expression of CAMs on the surfaces of both leukocytes and endothelial cells; hence, they can act to trigger or prolong the adhesion and emigration process.

The families of cell adhesion molecules are as follows:

Selectins: bind carbohydrates, initiate leukocyte-endothelial cell interactions

Integrins: bind to CAMs and extracellular matrix proteins, form strong adhesion

Immunoglobulin superfamily: members play various roles in cell adhesion

---

INFLAMMATORY MEDIATORS

Inflammatory mediators are secretory molecules produced by one cell that affect some function (chemotaxis, activation, or proliferation) of that same cell or an adjacent cell.

In addition to the cell contact-mediated stimulation of leukocytes, the state of activation of cells can be triggered by secretory products. These include cytokines (Table 10-2; Appendix 2), arachidonic acid metabolites (prostaglandins, leukotrienes, and thromboxanes) (Fig. 10-4), reactive nitrogen intermediates (nitric oxide), reactive oxygen intermediates (superoxide, hydroxyl radical, and hydrogen peroxide), histamine, and complement components.

Histamine is the major preformed mediator of mast cells (see Fig. 10-3). Formed from the amino acid histidine by an enzyme found in the cytoplasm of mast cells and basophils, its effects are mediated by two distinct classes of receptors, designated H_1 and H_2. Acute vascular inflammatory effects are transduced through H_1 receptors on the surfaces of smooth muscle cells, and the anti-inflammatory effects involve H_2 receptors.

The synthesis of nitric oxide takes place as follows:

$$\text{Arginine} \xrightarrow{\text{Nitric oxide synthase}} \text{Citrulline} + \text{Nitric oxide}$$

TABLE 10-2
KEY INFLAMMATORY CYTOKINES

CYTOKINE	MAJOR EFFECTS
Interleukin-1 (IL-1)	Activates endothelium and leukocytes, stimulates acute phase protein synthesis, fever
Interleukin-6 (IL-6)	Activates lymphocytes, increases antibody production, stimulates acute phase protein synthesis, fever
Interleukin-8 (IL-8)	Chemotactic for leukocytes (primarily neutrophils)
Interleukin-10 (IL-10)	Deactivates macrophages
Interleukin-12 (IL-12)	Activates lymphocytes, increases antibody production
Tumor necrosis factor α (TNFα)	Activates endothelium and increases permeability, fever, shock
Transforming growth factor β (TGFβ)	Deactivates macrophages, stimulates fibroblast collagen
Platelet-derived growth factor (PDGF)	Stimulates fibroblast proliferation

Nitric oxide and reactive oxygen intermediates could be thought of as secretory mediators, because they are made by one cell and exhibit their effects on another. The production of reactive nitrogen intermediates by mammalian cells is a recent observation, while the generation of reactive metabolites of oxygen has been known for some time. The oxygen intermediates include superoxide, hydroxyl radical, and hydrogen peroxide. Nitric oxide, which is synthesized from

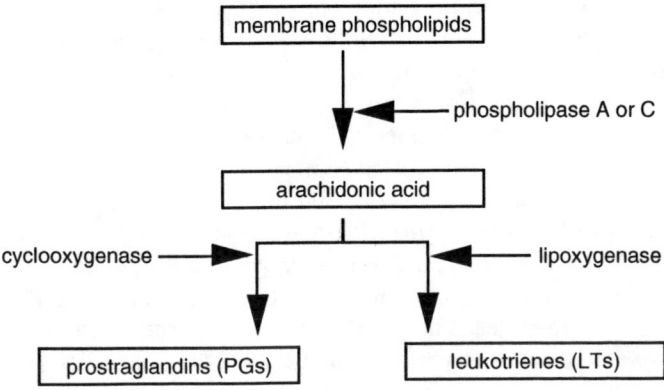

Figure 10-4
Arachidonic acid metabolism.

L-arginine in macrophages, appears to play a critical role in the antimicrobial activity. Nitric oxide synthase, the enzyme responsible for the production of the reactive intermediate, is activated by both cytokines (see Table 10-2) and microbial products.

CHRONIC INFLAMMATION

This is an inflammatory process that continues past the first few days.

When the infiltration of neutrophils is not sufficient to clear an inflamed area, then additional support is provided by non-granular leukocytes, lymphocytes, and macrophages. This marks the entry into *chronic inflammation*, which is of longer duration and involves several different types of cells that reside in the blood and the connective tissue.

Following are some cells of the monocyte/macrophage lineage:

Blood: monocytes
Connective tissue: macrophages
Lung: pulmonary or alveolar macrophages
Liver: Kupffer cells
Skin: Langerhans cells

Monocytes, the circulating precursor of tissue macrophages, remain in the circulation for 1 to 2 days prior to differentiation into *macrophages*. Macrophages are long-lived, highly motile, phagocytic cells that serve to protect tissue from foreign materials by internalizing (phagocytosis) and digesting it. Their cytoplasm contains large numbers of lysosomes and endocytic vacuoles and intracellular vesicles containing undigestible material. Under certain conditions, such as the invasion of foreign material, macrophages can form multinucleated giant cells, which result from the fusion of several macrophages. In addition to directed and random movement of the entire cell, macrophages can extend pseudopods in an ameboid fashion to reach out and explore their environment. Macrophages are also highly secretory cells that produce a variety of mediators, which range from cytokines and prostaglandins to connective tissue elements.

The return to normal tissue structure and function following a local inflammatory event depends on the degree of damage to the tissue and the ability of cells within the tissue to regenerate. Since at many inflammatory sites the epithelium is damaged, the resolution can be thought of as a "competition" between *reepithelialization*, which leads to a return to normal tissue structure and function, and *fibrosis*, the replacement of normal tissue with connective tissue containing fibroblasts and collagen. Evidence suggests that macrophages, as well as lymphocytes, play critical roles in both processes by elaborating cytokines, which enhance replication of epithelial cells and stimulate the proliferation of fibro-blasts (PDGF and IL-1) and the synthesis of extracellular matrix proteins, pri-marily type I collagen (TGFβ). In the absence of inhibitory signals, the aberrant production of these fibrogenic mediators sustains the connective tissue accumu-lation, resulting in permanent alteration in tissue architecture. While anti-inflam-matory and immunosuppressive agents, including glucocorticoids, have been used clinically to turn off the inflammatory cascade of events, these treatments cannot reverse the fibrotic process once it has been initiated.

ANATOMICAL LOCATION OF IMMUNE RESPONSES

•

- **Lymphocyte Migration into Lymphoid Tissues**
- **Germinal Centers**
- **Follicular Dendritic Cells**
- **Mucosal Immune System**

•   •   •   •   •   •   •   •   •   •   •   •   •

LYMPHOCYTE MIGRATION INTO LYMPHOID TISSUES

Lymphocyte migration into lymphoid tissues involves a family of adhesion molecules called *selectins*, *integrins*, and members of the *immunoglobin superfamily*.

As discussed in Chap. 2, both naive and memory lymphocytes continue to recirculate between blood and secondary lymphoid tissue. However, once activated, memory cells tend to recirculate back to the tissue where they were activated. As discussed in Chap. 10, lymphocytes respond to chemotactic signals from inflamed tissues or secondary lymphoid organs initially via surface glycoproteins called selectins. E-selectin (ELAM-1) on endothelial cells binds L-selectin (LAM-1) on lymphocytes, causing a loose association or *tethering*. Firm *adhesion* is mediated by lymphocyte *integrin* proteins such as VLA-4 or LFA-1 interacting with their respective ligand VCAM or ICAM (member of the immunoglobin superfamily) on the surface of endothelial cells. This adhesive interaction causes an activation of the lymphocyte to increase expression of integrin molecules, thus strengthening the adhesion. The endothelial cell then directs the lymphocyte toward its basal lamina while simultaneously down-regulating

ICAM expression. Migrating lymphocytes finally diapedese between endothelial cells into an organ or tissue by up-regulating production of proteinases.

Once a naive lymphocyte is activated, it displays a different density of adhesion molecules specific for the tissue in which it was initially activated, thus allowing it to repeatedly return to that tissue.

GERMINAL CENTERS

Germinal centers (GCs) develop within primary follicles of lymph nodes and spleen during T cell-dependent immune responses. GCs are the sites of centroblast clonal expansion and V_H region-directed somatic hypermutation, selection of high affinity antibody-producing centrocytes, deletion of low affinity centrocytes, Th1- and Th2-directed antibody class isotype production and eventual generation of plasmablasts or memory cells (see Fig. 11-1).

B cells in lymph nodes and spleen first encounter Ag in the T cell-rich areas of the paracortex and periarterial lymphoid sheath (PALS), respectively. Ag is presented to them by dendritic cells (DCs), which express high levels of class II major histocompatibility complex (MHC), adhesion, and co-stimulatory molecules. After activation, and within 2 days, these B blasts produce low affinity unmutated Ig, which is capable of forming Ag-Ig complexes on follicular dendritic cells within primary follicles. Many of these cells die within 10 to 12 days. On the average, three B blasts colonize each primary follicle and are then called *centroblasts*. Centroblasts, which are found in the base or dark zone of the follicle, down-regulate their surface Ig and undergo a clonal expansion phase, dividing every 6 to 7 h. During proliferation, they activate a site-specific hypermutation mechanism that introduces random point mutations into their Ig V_H region genes. *Centrocytes* are the progeny of centroblasts that migrate apically into the basal light zone, where they up-regulate their somatically mutated surface Ig (receptors). Here, they interact with follicular dendritic cells (FDCs), which can contain unprocessed Ag in the form of immune (Ag-Ab) complexes on their surface for months. The centrocytes that express somatically mutated surface Ig receptors with high (↑) affinity for FDC-bound Ag up-regulate bcl-2 expression and are positively selected (which is opposite to positive selection of thymocytes (Chap. 5)). These centrocytes interact with Th_2 cells and can become either plasmablasts or memory B cells, depending on the co-stimulatory signals they receive from FDC and Th1 or Th2 cells. However, they also have a high propensity to recycle back into centroblasts for further proliferation and even higher affinity maturation. Centrocytes with low affinity somatically mutated surface Ig (receptors) for FDC-Ag do not up-regulate bcl-2 and die via apoptosis (see Fig. 14-2). Thus, there is extensive fine tuning of centrocytes before they are allowed to produce antibody for export.

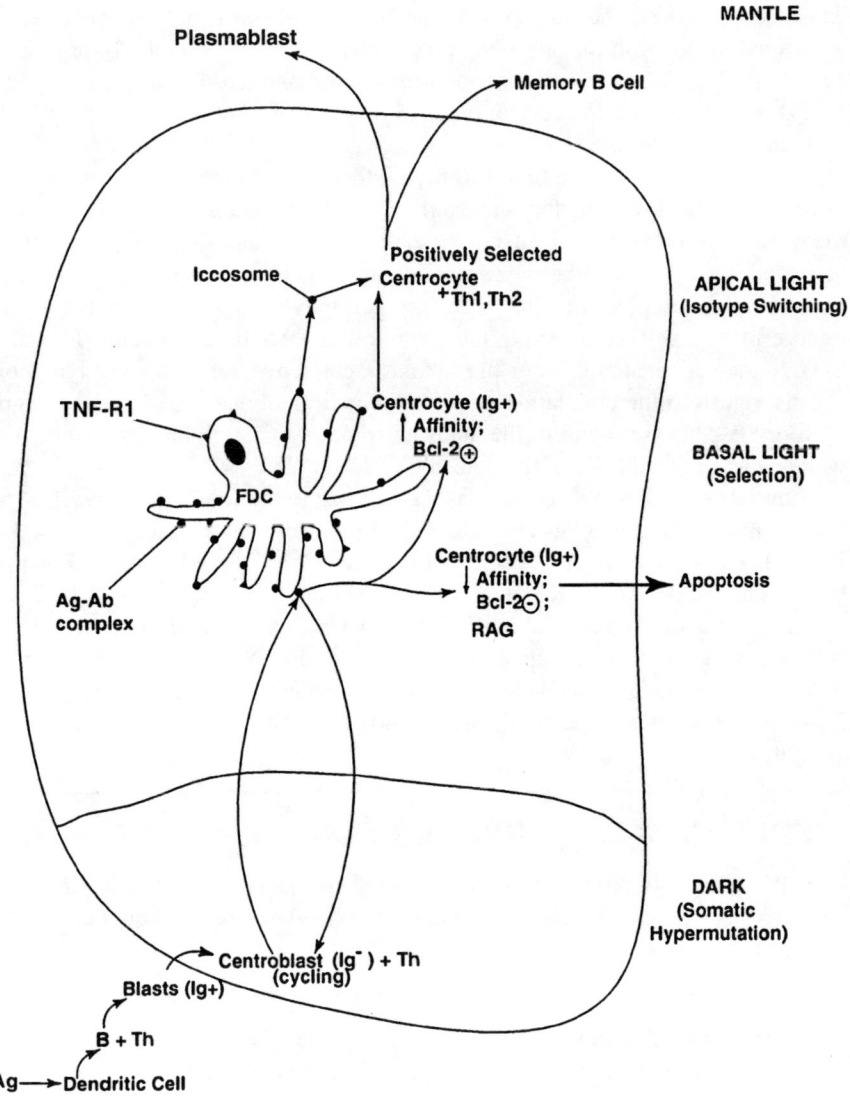

Figure 11-1
GC zones.

The recombination-activating genes *RAG*1 and *RAG*2, which drive genomic V(D)J rearrangements (described in Chap. 4 during development of B cells in the bone marrow) are also induced to be reexpressed in preapoptotic centrocytes of the basal light zone. This induction of an immature state in GC centrocytes may be necessary for further light chain receptor editing in an effort to save these cells.

This editing of V_L genes, along with the bcl-2-regulated apoptosis, provides an additional mechanism for removing potentially autoreactive antibody-producing cells. Thus, in GC, there is an opportunity for antigen-dependent secondary V(D)J rearrangements to occur in order to fine tune the specificity of the peripheral antibody repertoire.

Once centrocytes with high affinity surface Ig and high expression of bcl-2 have passed the discriminatory environment of the basal light zone, they migrate to the apical light zone. Here Ab class switching and maturation into plasmablasts or memory cells occur. Plasmablasts migrate into the medullary cords of lymph nodes and red pulp cord of the spleen, where they terminally differentiate into mature plasma cells and secrete their antibodies into the circulation (Figs 2-2, 2-3). Some activated B cells or plasmablasts can leave the secondary lymphoid organs, return to the circulation, and reappear in the bone marrow and the gut. Memory B cells are found in the areas surrounding GCs (follicular mantles) as well as the marginal zone of the spleen (see Chap. 2).

Initial proliferation of centroblasts gives rise to the first foci in primary follicles within 2 days, and the development of a full dark and light zone GC takes 14 days. The development of GCs requires cluster formation between LFA-1 on B cells and ICAM-1 on FDCs as well as VLA-4 on activated B cells and VCAM on FDCs. In addition, interleukin-4, -5, and -10 must be elicited from Th1 or Th2 cells in order for antibody class switching and full centrocyte development to plasmablasts or memory cells to occur. GCs in spleen and lymph nodes peak at 2 weeks and begin to wane after 3 weeks; however, GCs remain constitutively in the gut.

FOLLICULAR DENDRITIC CELLS

FDCs have long processes and Fc, C, TNF receptors, as well as ICAM-1, and VCAM-1 but no MHC-II. They contain Ag-Ab complexes on their surface for months to years.

Centrocytes that continue to maintain high levels of bcl-2 expression can receive membrane-bound immune complexes (iccosomes) from FDC and induce the expression of T cell-reactive surface molecules such as B7.2. This resultant interaction determines whether there is differentiation into a mature GC centrocyte or centroblast recycling. However, the formation of FDC clusters is critically dependent on TNFα and LTα, since these cytokines are necessary for FDC cluster formation and consequent primary as well as secondary follicles indicating that they have TNF-R1s.

The fact that FDC can contain Ag for prolonged periods of time is the reason why we do not need to be frequently immunized with certain antigens, since FDCs provide a continuous depot of Ag even without an existing GC. It has recently been recognized that the human immunodeficiency virus, upon disappearing from the blood, can be sequestered on the dendritic arms of FDC for a number of years. Eventually, the FDC can no longer hold the virus in check, the virus is released into peripheral blood, and the patient enters the lethal stages of AIDS.

MUCOSAL IMMUNE SYSTEM

The *mucosal immune system* (MIS) consists of lymphoid tissues within and directly beneath the epithelial lining of the respiratory, genitourinary, and gastrointestinal tracts as well as beneath the ductal system of the salivary, lacrimal, and mammary glands. The surface area of mucosal surfaces is over 100 times greater than that of skin, and the MIS contains up to 75% of all the B cells of the body. The primary product of the MIS is IgA.

Within the gastrointestinal tract, soluble antigen is taken up by villus epithelium and particulate antigens are primarily taken up in the ileal portion of the small intestine by specialized surface lining microfold (M) cells (Fig. 11-2). M cells internalize Ag and transport it to underlying lamina propria macrophages,

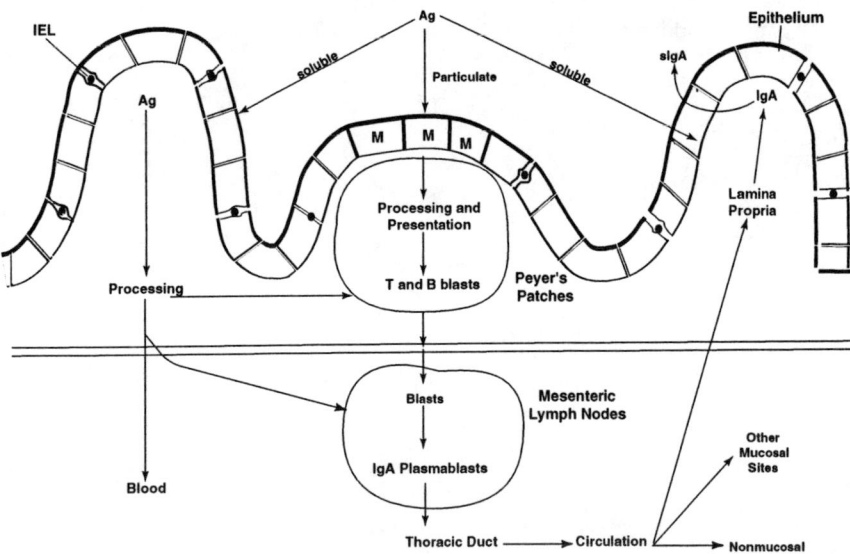

Figure 11-2
Ag and cell traffic in gut.

which process it and present it to surrounding collections of lymphoid cells forming ileal Peyer's patches (PPs). PPs contain follicles, similar to lymph nodes and spleen, with high endothelial venules and significant collections of T cells in between. T and B blasts activated here go to the nearest mesenteric lymph node for further maturation, alpha H chain class switching, or J chain formation or deletion. They then enter the thoracic duct and bloodstream, homing back to the same or distant mucosal sites. Thus, even though much of the processing and reactivity to antigen occurs in the ileum, protection through IgA occurs at many mucosal surfaces.

Serum IgA is monmeric and represents only 11% of all serum immunoglobulin. Secretory IgA represents over 95% of all Ig found in secretions and is primarily dimeric with two monomeric units covalently joined by a J chain. Dimeric IgA binds to a polymeric immunoglobulin receptor (pIGR) on the basal surface of mucosal epithelial cells. This IgA-pIGR complex is endocytosed and transported to the apical (luminal) surface of the epithelial cell. During this transport process, a small piece of the pIGR is cleaved with the remaining component now called the *secretory component*. Thus, IgA is secreted as dimeric IgA bound to a secretory component.

Secretory IgA does not activate the complement system but coats bacteria and some viruses (polio, coxsackie, rota, and herpes), thus preventing their adherence to mucosal lining epithelium. Also, some viruses within surface epithelia can be neutralized by pIGR-internalized IgA. However, it should be noted that oral immunization with soluble Ag does not always generate an immune response and can instead generate unresponsiveness.

IMMEDIATE
HYPERSENSITIVITY

•

•　•　•　•　•　•　•　•　•　•　•　•

ALLERGIC RESPONSE

An allergic response occurs when the host is reexposed to an antigen that it has encountered previously.

Any allergic symptoms that occur within the exposed individual are not caused by the antigen but are caused by the immune products that are released from immune cells that recognize and react against the invading antigen. The mechanism most responsible for immediate allergic reactions involves the production of antibodies by B cells and of cytokines by T cells. As discussed in Chap. 3, antibodies are made against any hapten carrier protein complex (e.g., inhaled particulates, such as ragweed pollen). The subsequent antibody response that develops against this antigen is specific for the hapten, even though the carrier protein is important for the stimulation of cytokine production by CD4+ T cells that will help B cells make the antibody. Also, local presentation of antigen (e.g., in the skin) induces the release of inflammatory cytokines from T cells that precipitate a local inflammatory response.

Allergic responses have been categorized into four groups, depending on the nature of the immunologic reaction.

ALLERGIC RESPONSE TYPES

Group I responses involve the production of IgE antibodies that trigger the release of substances from mast cells that trigger anaphylaxis and allergic rhinitis.

Group II responses involve primarily IgG antibodies that attach to a cell surface, react with complement, and cause cell lysis.

Group III responses involve primarily IgG antibodies that form complexes with antigen and complement to recruit phagocytic cells such as neutrophils to a site where they can release inflammatory cytokines, which will result in local inflammation.

Group IV responses involve sensitized T cells that release inflammatory cytokines that induce allergic contact dermatitis.

Group I allergic responses induce the most prevalent chronic discomfort symptoms for many individuals. Hay fever is included in this group. As shown in Fig. 12-1, when pollen grains enter an individual's respiratory tract, they are transported to a local lymph node that makes up the bronchiole-associated lymphoid tissue. The antigen is then recognized by a B cell immunoglobulin receptor. The B cell processes this antigen and presents it to Th cells, an event that activates the Th cell to make cytokines. If a Th2 cell type is activated, the cell will produce interleukin-4 (see Fig. 13-2). Interleukin-4 is required for the B cell to produce IgE antibodies, which then bind to a special Fc receptor located on mast cells residing within the respiratory epithelium of the nasal and bronchiolar cavities. When pollen reenters the respiratory tract, it binds to the immunoglobulin receptor of the IgE antibody attached to the mast cell, resulting in the release of histamine from the mast cell. As described in Chap. 10, histamine induces the classical symptoms of hay fever, namely bronchial constriction, edema of the nasal mucosa, increased mucus production, and inflammation of the respiratory tract itself. Antihistamines relieve these symptoms.

Clinical syndromes induced by IgE-mediated allergic reactions

allergic rhinitis: inhaled antigen (pollen) → edema and irritation of nasal mucosa

bronchial asthma: inhaled antigen (pollen) → bronchial constriction, increased mucus

systemic anaphylaxis: intravenous antigen (drugs or venom) → vasodilation, edema, tracheal occlusion, death

wheal and flare: skin antigen (insect bite) → localized vasodilation and swelling

food allergy: ingested antigen (milk) → vomiting and diarrhea

---

The clinical syndromes that exemplify the above example of an allergic reaction mediated by IgE antibodies are *allergic rhinitis* and *bronchial asthma*. Systemic anaphylaxis is another clinical syndrome that involves an IgE-mediated allergic response. In contrast to allergic rhinitis and bronchial asthma that involve a localized reaction to antigen, *systemic anaphylaxis* involves a reaction to antigen that has disseminated throughout the body via the bloodstream. In this case, the antigen binds to IgE bound to mast cells located in the connective tissue of all blood vessels in the body. The symptoms resulting from the disseminated release of histamine include vasodilation, edema, occlusion of the trachea, and death. Two other clinical syndromes that involve an allergic reaction mediated by IgE antibodies include the *wheal and flare* syndrome, which is induced by allergen skin testing and insect bites to produce a local vasodilation and edema, and the *food allergy* syndrome, which is induced by food products to induce a severe response by mast cells residing within the connective tissue of the gut that results in transepithelial fluid loss and smooth muscle contraction, resulting in vomiting and diarrhea.

Group II and III allergic responses involve primarily IgG antibody but do not involve the release of histamine from mast cells. Thus, in contrast to IgE-mediated allergic responses that occur in a matter of seconds, IgG-mediated allergic responses occur within a few hours of antigen exposure. *Group II allergic responses* involve the binding of IgG antibodies to antigens that are expressed on the surface of cells residing in the body (Fig. 12-2). For example, some drugs affix to cells in the body, such as red blood cells. Circulating IgG antibodies that recognize the drug bind to the antigen bound to the cell. As described in Chap. 14, the cell-bound IgG activates complement and Fcγ receptor-bearing cells, such as macrophages and neutrophils, as it would in the defense reaction against microorganisms. In this manner, healthy cells of the body are lysed and destroyed.

Group III allergic responses involve primarily IgG antibody that binds to soluble antigens found in either the circulation or extracellular fluid. In the skin, the IgG antibody and antigen form insoluble complexes that activate complement to produce inflammatory mediators (e.g., C5a) that increase vascular permeability and attract neutrophils to the site of the immune complexes (Fig. 12-3). The neutrophils then phagocytose the complexes and eliminate them from the site. However, some antibody-antigen complexes circulate and deposit themselves on Fcγ receptor-bearing cells of the vasculature, kidney, lungs, and joints. The IgG portion of the complexes activates complement and phagocytes, resulting in considerable tissue damage that results in clinical diseases such as vasculitis, nephritis and arthritis.

Group IV allergic responses are primarily mediated by soluble molecules that are released by specifically activated T cells. These are the delayed type hypersensitivity reactions that are the topic of Chap. 13.

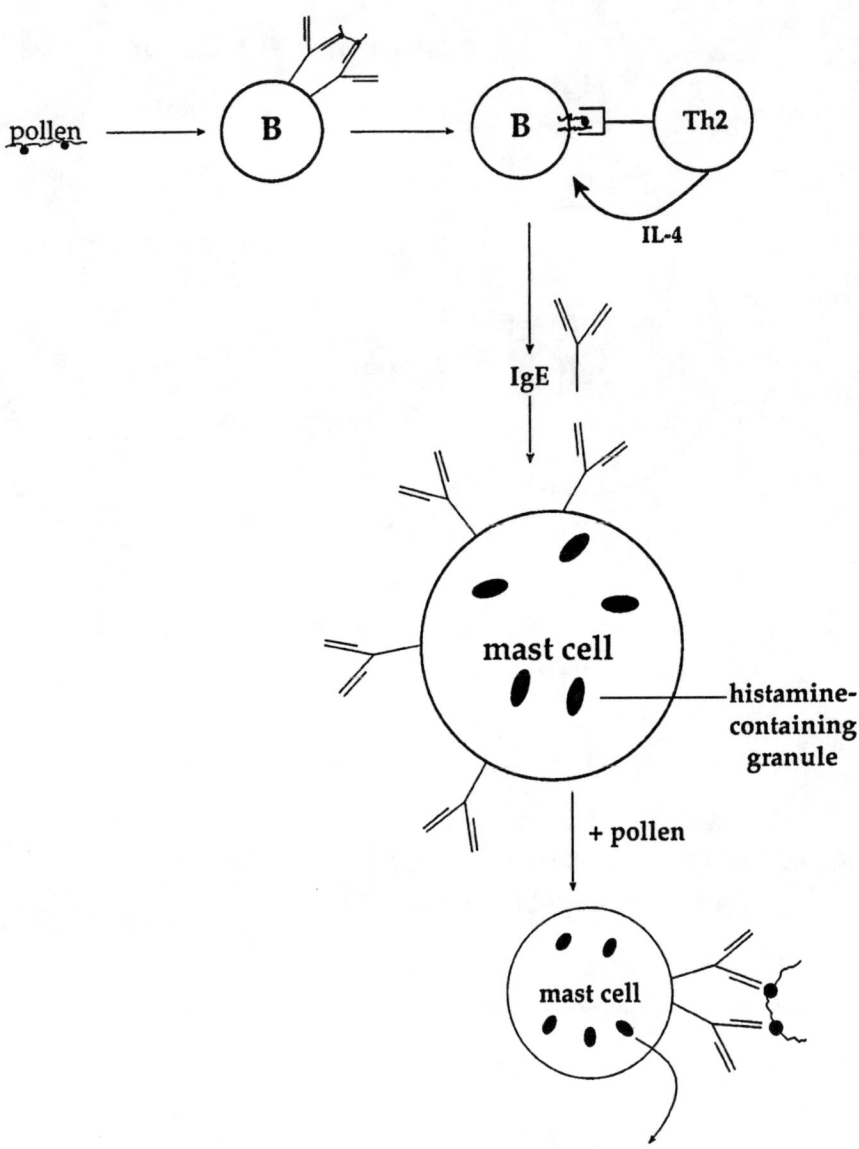

Figure 12-1
IgE-mediated allergic response.

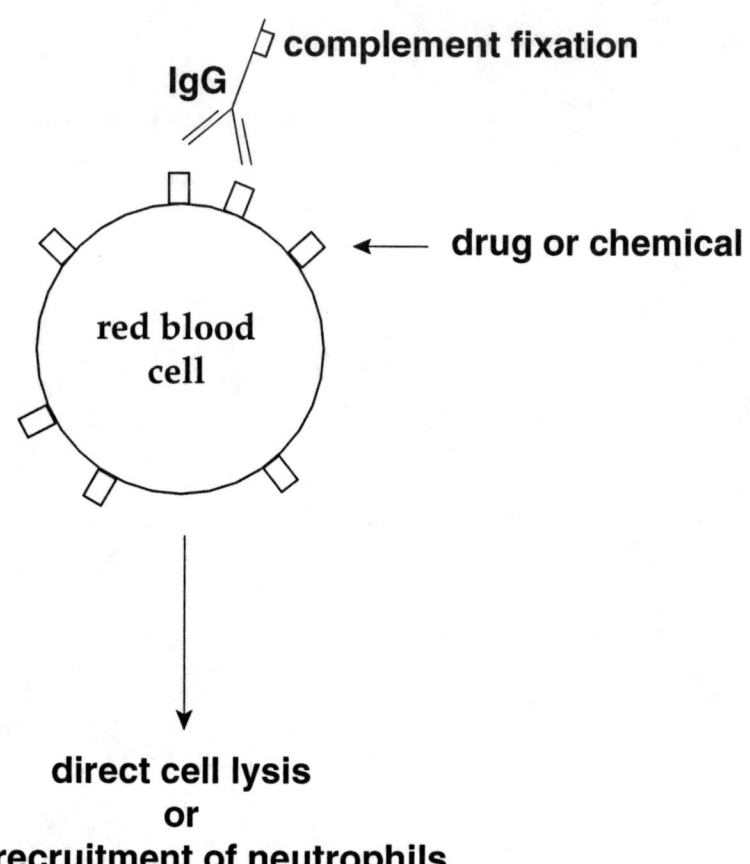

Figure 12-2
IgG-mediated allergic response to insoluble antigens.

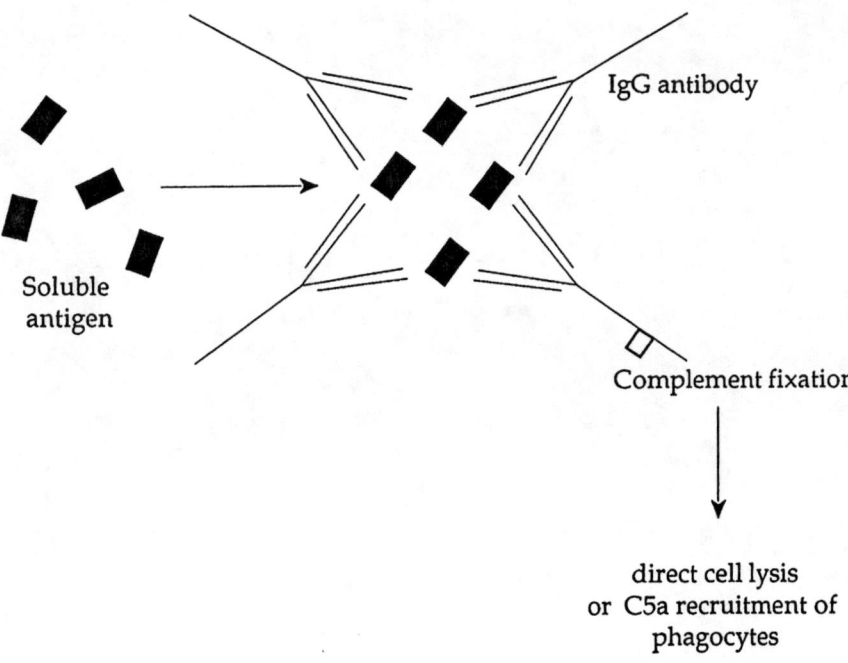

Figure 12-3
IgG-mediated allergic response to soluble antigens.

DELAYED TYPE HYPERSENSITIVITY (DTH)

·

- **Cell-mediated Immunity (CMI)**
- **T Cell Subsets**
- **Cytokines and CMI**
- **Cytokines and Th Subsets**
- **Interferon-γ**
- **Induction of DTH**
- **Proinflammatory Component of DTH**
- **Antigen-specific Component of DTH**
- **Regulation of DTH**

· · · · · · · · · · · ·

CELL-MEDIATED IMMUNITY

Cell-mediated immunity is the ability of T cells to recognize major histocompatibility complex (MHC)-presented antigens, become activated, and produce and react to cytokines. Depending upon the type of T cell activated, either antigen-specific or macrophage-mediated cytotoxicity ensues.

As you have learned from previous chapters, T cells are the primary orchestrators and mediators of immune responses. The escalating complexity of external threats to host survival exemplified by viruses and pathogenic bacteria, coupled with the parallel need for intensified internal surveillance mechanisms of diversified body and cell structure, forced T cells to devise new, specific, and focused host defense strategies. *Cell-mediated immunity* has developed along two pathways, both of which are dependent upon precise recognition of altered host cells by the constant surveillance and sampling of peptides nestled in the MHC complex on nucleated cell surfaces (see Chap. 6) by T cells. Host cells that display altered MHC class I peptide complexes arising after viral infection or by generation of neoproteins by tumor genes provide a highly specific alerting mechanism that initiates the differentiation of CD3$^+$8$^+$ T cells to highly effective cytolytic or killer T cells (CTLs). The cytotoxic mechanisms used by CTLs are discussed in Chap. 14.

The other major form of antigen-specific T cell-mediated immunity is *delayed type hypersensitivity (DTH)*. Although a better description of this defensive reaction might be T cell-mediated monocyte/macrophage (M/M) activation, the term DTH is firmly entrenched in both the experimental and clinical literature. In reality, DTH is delayed only in the sense that a time lag occurs between antigen-specific T lymphocyte stimulation and its subsequent recruitment and activation of a critical mass of effector macrophages to cope with the pathogen. A fundamental difference between DTH and CTL responses is that DTH reactions are set in motion by T cell recognition of peptide antigens displayed in the binding site of an MHC class II, not class I molecule (Fig. 13-1).

Although crude *in vivo* and *in vitro* assays of DTH have been available to researchers for years, the milestone discovery of T helper (Th) cell subsets provided the theoretical basis for our understanding of the dynamics of a DTH reaction.

T CELL SUBSETS

Thymocytes that successfully emigrate from the thymus as mature T cells (see Chap. 5) can be phenotypically divided into two major subgroups, CD3$^+$8$^+$ CTL cytolytic precursors and CD3$^+$CD4$^+$ helper cells. There are 2 times more CD4$^+$ T cells circulating in the peripheral blood under normal conditions than CD8$^+$ T cells.

The first inkling that CD3$^+$CD4$^+$ cells had disparate, indeed competing or polarized, functions arose during studies with well characterized mouse T helper cell lymphocyte clones. Similar functional differences in human CD4 lymphocytes were initially difficult to document and strongly contested, but now the presence of CD4 subsets in humans is universally accepted.

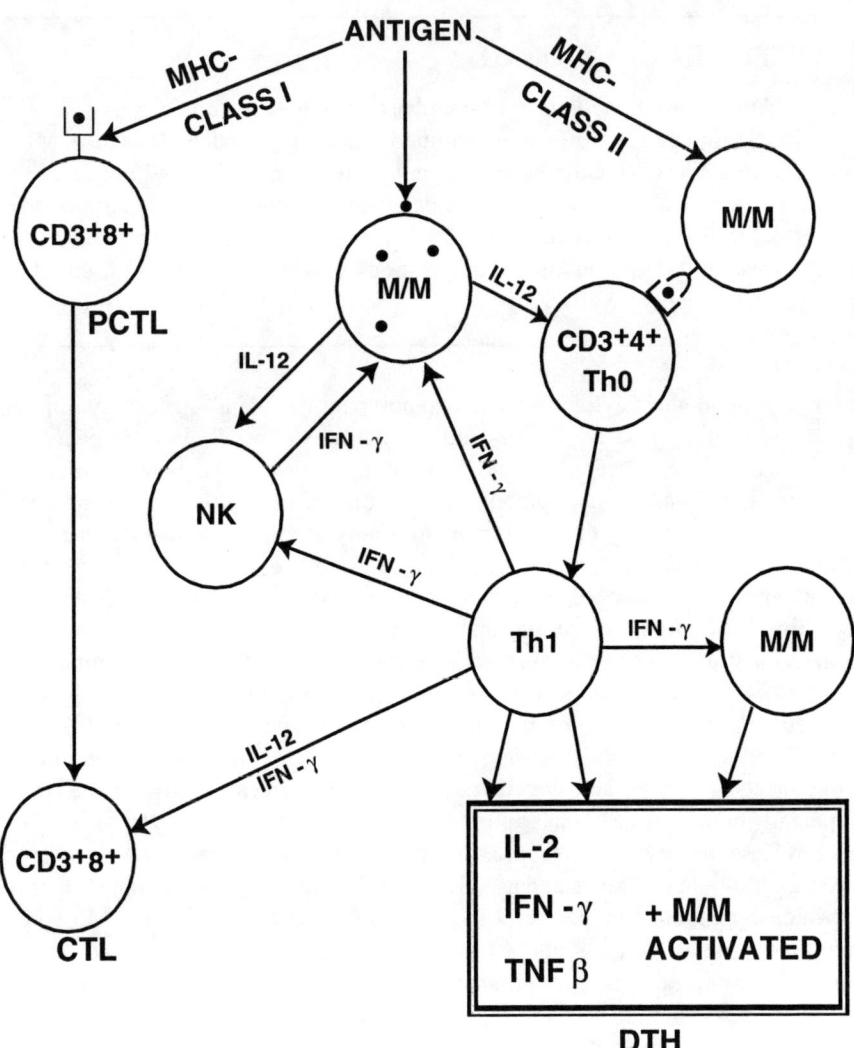

Figure 13-1
Cell-mediated immunity.

CYTOKINES AND CMI

Cytokines are *the mediators* of cellular communications that provide the critical signals for effective humoral (antibody-mediated) and CMI responses. $CD4^+$ T cells have antigen-specific amplifying and regulatory functions that are critical to the maintenance of immunologic homeostasis. CD4 T cells are subdivided into Th1 helper cells and Th2 helper cells on the basis of their production of and responses to specific *cytokines*, not by standard phenotypic differences.

In general, most cytokines have two polypeptide chains encoded by separate genes. Homology studies strongly suggest that most "new" cytokine genes and the genes for their receptors have evolved from primordial hemoproliferative growth factors and immunoglobulin gene clusters by duplication events. This concept is supported by the *overlapping* of many of their biologic effects. Evolutionary pressures have driven most cytokine systems to develop pleiotropism and redundancy. For example, fish and even worms produce some of the same cytokines that humans do during immune responses. Cytokines act at concentrations similar to endocrine hormones, are homo- or heterodimer polypeptides with a 70–190-amino acid composition, and are usually produced only after appropriate cell stimuli. They are *not* in themselves antigen-specific but can and do arise after T and/or B cell *antigen-specific activation*. That is, antigen-specific immune effector cells, T cells and B cells, and their non-antigen-specific counterparts, especially monocytes and macrophages, "talk" to each other via cytokine production, release, and cytokine receptor display. Both lymphocytes and macrophages produce multiple cytokines and use them to either *dampen* or *accentuate* the level of intensity of an immune response (i.e., regulate the response). Most cell-cytokine systems have agonist/antagonist (yin-yang) dynamics in order to prevent *runaway reactions*, and immune effector cells use cytokines to "fine tune" their responses, not only by varying the type and amount of cytokine production but also by regulating the density and affinity of cytokine receptors. Even if excess cytokines are released during an exuberant immune response, down-regulation of their receptors on their target cell surfaces will prevent a self-destructive immune reaction (Fig. 13-2).

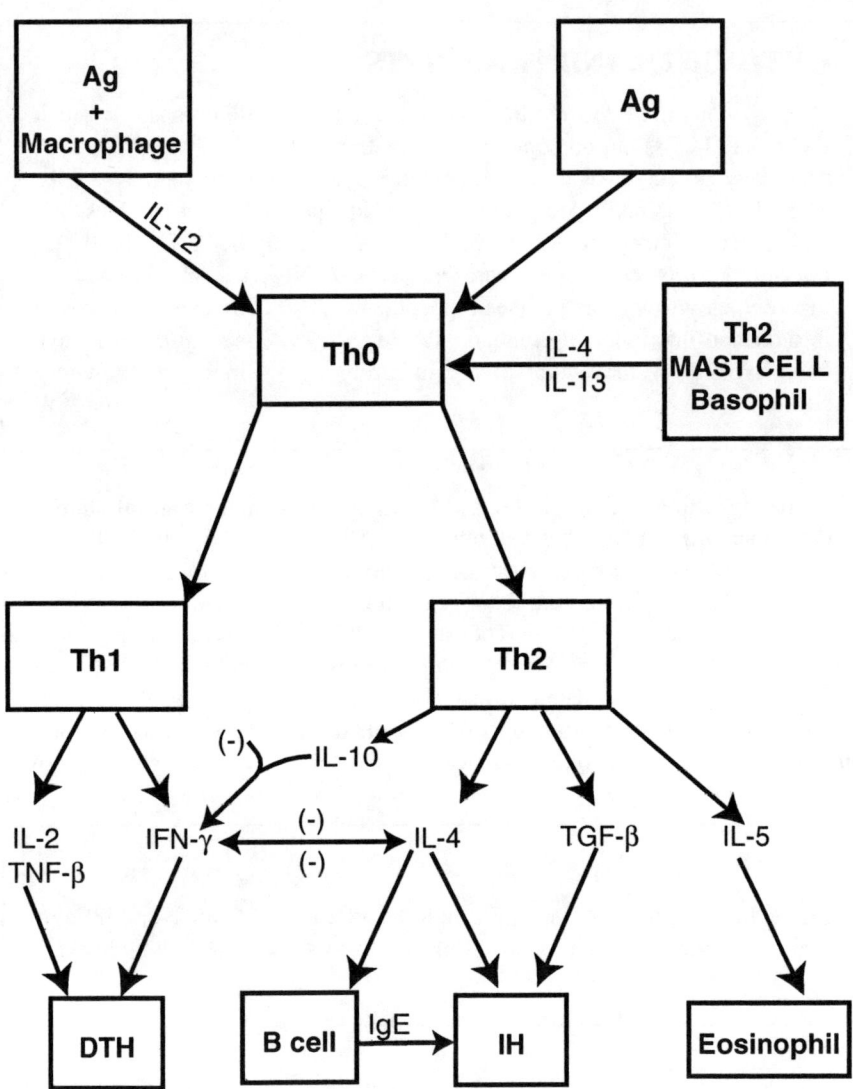

Figure 13-2
Development of Th1 and Th2 functions.

CYTOKINES AND Th SUBSETS

CD4$^+$ T cells migrate from the thymus armed with antigen-specific T cell receptors (TCRs) but no commitment to either the CD4$^+$ Th1 or Th2 subset. These precursor or naive CD4 lymphocytes are designated Th0 cells. They have a genetic pedigree for a broad spectrum of cytokines that includes interleukin (IL)-2, IL-3, IL-4, IL-5, IL-6, IL-9, IL-10, IL-13, interferon (IFN)-γ, tumor necrosis factor (TNF-β), and granulocyte/macrophage growth factors (see Appendix 2). Th0 cells can be provoked into further functional differentiation by *specific cytokine profiles* that have been evoked by the nature of the infecting organism or inflammatory stimulus.

The signature cytokine in the local microenvironment of an inflammatory reaction that will initiate the development of Th1 cells from precursor Th0 is IL-12. *IL-12* is the *critical early activating (initiation) cytokine* of DTH. This M/M cytokine is also a vigorous stimulator of natural killer (NK) cell proliferation and subsequent production of *IFN-γ*. The latter cytokine initiates amplifying immune and inflammatory reactions by activating additional NK cells and M/Ms, which then release more IL-12. The end result is commitment of Th0 cells to the Th1 subset. IFN-γ, a strong promoter of Th1 cell development, is also the *major inhibitor* of Th0 cells becoming Th2 cells.

INTERFERON-γ

IFN-γ has a central and pivotal role in all phases of immune and inflammatory responses. It is produced only by CD4 subset (Th1) lymphocytes and NK cells.

Once committed, Th1 cells can then be identified by their production of IL-2, IFN-γ, and TNF-β, also known as lymphotoxin (LTα) (Table 13-1; Appendix 2).

Conversely, if the cytokine milieu encountered by Th0 precursors is characterized predominately by *IL-4* and *IL-13*, Th0 cells become committed to Th2 cell differentiation. IL-4 is the *major agonist/growth factor* for the Th2 lymphocyte subset and a major promotor of humoral antibody responses. It is a *major antagonist* of Th1 subset development. IL-4 has potent effects on the growth and differentiation characteristics of B lymphocytes and is an isotype switch promoter that induces IgM-producing B cells to further differentiation and synthesis of IgG. It is an *absolute* requirement for an IgE response to parasites and other anti-

TABLE 13-1
CYTOKINE PROFILES OF CD3$^+$4$^+$ T CELLS

	Th0	Th1	Th2
IL-2	+	++	−
INF-γ	+	++	−
TNF-β	+	++	−
IL-4	+	−	++
IL-5	+	−	++
IL-10	+	−	++
IL-13	+	−	++

gen-specific IgE (allergic) responses or immediate hypersensitivity (IH). IL-4 and -13 have a very similar ancestry and structural homologies that are reflected in their redundant and overlapping biologic activities. *IL-10* is an especially important counterregulatory cytokine. IL-10 is a member of the four-α-helix cytokine family and an 18-kD polypeptide that is produced relatively "late" in an ongoing immune response by activated Th2 cells and M/M. Like IL-4, it is another *major antagonist* of DTH responses generated by Th1, NK cells, and M/M. Th2 cells can therefore also be characterized by their reaction to and production of a specific group of cytokines, IL-4, -5, -10 and -13 (Table 13-1). The functions of the two Th subsets and their cytokine counterparts are polarized and can be visualized as functioning in counterregulatory relationships (Table 13-2 and Fig. 13-2). Th1 responses, while highly effective in most instances against many forms of intracellular infections, can cause wide spread tissue damage if allowed to run rampant. Th2 responses have developed strategies to attenuate ongoing DTH reactions as they simultaneously promote specific antibody responses important for the prevention of disseminated infection. This is important, since certain infections require Th1 cytokines for their resolution (tuberculosis, leprosy, and others) but other infections (e.g., parasitic infections) require Th2 cytokines for resolution and the presence of Th1 cytokines may be extremely detrimental in terminating them. Thus, interference with or defects in the delicate balance between CD4 Th1 and Th2 subsets or their cytokine production and receptor display have important implications for the manifestations of many diseases.

INDUCTION OF DTH

Antigen-specific DTH responses develop in response to specific types of infection.

The complex interactions of cytokines and effector cells that culminate in DTH begin when polysaccharide cell wall components of a pathogen are recognized in a innate or non-antigen-specific manner by macrophages. Certain pathogens, even though internalized, successfully evade killing by macrophage lytic and oxidative mechanisms. When macrophages are unable to resist infection with their innate defense mechanisms, they must invoke more effective cell-mediated immunity. They do so by driving Th0 differentiation of cells to Th1 and thereby initiating DTH. After intercellular infection with a DTH-evoking pathogen, M/M turn on their antigen-presenting function to modify and process microbial antigens in their cytoplasm, link them on site to the MHC class II molecules, and then transport the MHC-antigen complex to the cell surface, where their antigenic peptides are displayed in the class II MHC antigen binding site (see Chap. 7). Once specific CD4/TCR antigen binding and appropriate co-activation signals such as CD40/CD40L and CD28/B7 occur (see Chap. 8), a DTH reaction begins.

PROINFLAMMATORY COMPONENT OF DTH

Macrophages, in a nonspecific and early response to the intracellular infection, produce and release the *proinflammatory cytokines* IL-1, IL-6, and TNF-α. Proinflammatory cytokines have broad anti-inflammatory properties and stimulate generalized stress adaptations by organ systems such as liver and central nervous system; however, these are front-line, temporizing defenses that act to slow down the pace of an infection while more specific immune defenses are mobilized.

IL-1 has an extraordinarily large range of biological effects, many of which are not restricted to the immune system. IL-1 can be viewed as a *primordial cytokine* with broad spectrum effects that facilitate host reaction to stress and infection. IL-1 is produced by a wide range of cell types, especially M/M and keratinocytes, that respond to other cytokine stimuli and a wide diversity of microbial and environmental stimuli, including silica crystals and even certain UV wavelengths. It is a *cardinal proinflammatory mediator* that can elevate body temperature by its effects on the hypothalamus, stimulate synthesis (in concert with IL-6) of acute phase host protective proteins by the liver, mobilize neutrophils from the bone marrow, and induce colony-stimulating factors that accelerate the production of neutrophils and increase their mobilization. IL-1 also has neuroendocrine effects that act via the pituitary axis to release adrenocorticotrophic hormone, which increases the production of adrenal corticosteroids as a stress response. Critical in the early portion of immunologic reactions, IL-1 facilitates the activation of peripheral mature activated T cells and supports their proliferation by increasing IL-2 receptor display. IL-1, in *autocrine* fashion, also stimulates antigen-presenting cells to be more efficient antigen presenters.

IL-1ra is the naturally occurring antagonist of IL-1 and competes for IL-1 receptors. Clearly, it is synthesized to prevent the severe morbidity of an unbridled IL-1-driven inflammatory response. *IL-6* can be discussed in the same context as IL-1 in that IL-6 has many redundant, broad spectrum biologic effects characteristic of IL-1. IL-6 is also produced by a broad spectrum of cells, including T cells, monocytes, and fibroblasts. IL-6, in concert with IL-1, also induces IL-2 responsiveness in T cells and is a major requirement for T cell activation. Similar to almost all other cytokines, it is not produced until its cell source is provoked by initiating cytokines. A major *distinguishing* function from IL-1 is its effects on *B cell growth* and increased resistance to apoptosis. This B cell-nurturing quality has evoked clinical interest in the use of anti-IL-6 agents for the treatment of plasma cell proliferative disorders. Very recently, IL-6 has also been shown to have a strong influence on the development of mucosal immunity.

Another major mediator of defensive cellular responses is *TNF-α*, a cytokine polypeptide produced mainly by activated M/M (and other cells), with very broad and predominantly proinflammatory effects. IL-1 and TNF-α are almost indistinguishable in their biologic effects during an immunological reaction. The primordial significance of TNF-α is reflected by its gene location within the MHC complex. This cytokine is an extraordinarily potent *M/M activator* that confers the ability to kill antibody-coated target cells and increases M/M lytic and oxidative capabilities for killing bacteria viruses and parasites. *TNF-β* (also called lymphotoxin α), released by activated Th1 cells, is very closely related to the TNF-α in structure and function. One apparent unique feature of TNF-β is its influence on the development of lymph nodes and spleen. Mice that have the TNF-β gene deleted develop normal T and B cells and have a normal thymus but have abnormal peripheral lymphoid tissue, especially germinal centers.

ANTIGEN-SPECIFIC COMPONENT OF DTH

The antigen-specific DTH reaction begins when macrophage-derived IL-12, in concert with antigen presentation by M/M MHC class II, promotes Th0 commitment to the Th1 subset. A cardinal characteristic of DTH is that an activated antigen-specific Th1-helper cell can recruit massive numbers of non-antigen-specific but highly effective activated killer macrophages to the site of inflammation.

After Th0 commitment to the Th1 subset, the activated cell Th0 (soon to become a Th1 cell) rapidly increases IL-2 production, which stimulates, in the presence of IL-1, Th1 clonal expansion. *IL-2* is a major *initiation cytokine* and a *pivotal growth hormone* in the immune response. It is produced by activated Th cells, acts in an autocrine and paracrine fashion, and also enhances NK and B cell growth. IL-2 is a 15-kD glycoprotein, and its functional activities are dependent on an intact tertiary structure. The high affinity IL-2 receptor consists of three polypeptide chains in heterodimer form that are only expressed as a functional unit after specific antigen TCR interactions. One of the three IL-2 receptor chains is also an integral part of several other cytokines, especially IL-4 and IL-7. This is another example of cytokine redundancy that provides a fail-safe means of T cell growth. The pivotal role of IL-2 in an effective immune response makes it obvious that abnormalities or manipulations of this cytokine or its receptors should have clinical implications. Thus, genetic defects in the assembly of the IL-2 receptor have been shown to result in a severe immunodeficiency state.

IFN-γ, already present in increasing amounts from NK cells, but now also resulting from antigen-specific Th1 activation and proliferation, amplifies the DTH reaction by stimulating the display of endothelial adhesion molecules, which divert circulating macrophages, lymphocytes, and neutrophils to the area of inflammation (see Chaps. 10 and 11).

Exits and entries into and from the vascular distribution system are governed by a complex set of interacting recognition structures termed *adhesion molecules* or *selectins*.

The surveillance migration of T cells through peripheral lymph nodes is guided by adhesion/homing molecules on high endothelial venules (Chaps. 2 and 11). Efficient diversion and exit into areas of inflammation depends on the activation of a second set of adhesion/homing molecules on endothelium and local increased blood flow. L-selectins are expressed on leukocytes, P-selectins are found in the alpha granules of platelets, and E-selectins are found on endothelium. E-selectins provide a highly efficient mechanism for diverting immune effector cells to the site of an ongoing immunologic/inflammatory response, since they are displayed on endothelial cells *only after cytokine activation*. The sorting/diverting mechanism begins when activated adhesion molecules on the endothelium attract effector cells from the capillary mainstream and facilitate a rolling motion along endothelium cells. Once rolling on the endothelium occurs, there is increasingly frequent contact of lymphocyte receptors with these activated endothelial cell surface determinants. The effector cell is coaxed across the endothelial cell by a second set of adhesion molecules termed *ICAM-1* (CD54), *VCAM-1*, and *ECAM-1*. These adhesion molecules are genetic descendants of the immunoglobulin supergene family; are widely distributed on endothelium, epithelium, and fibroblast surfaces; and are capable of *rapid upregulation by cytokines* during an immune response and promote firm adhesion and transendothelial migration of immune effector cells to the site of the inflammatory stimulus.

A mandatory participant for a fully developed DTH reaction is IFN-γ. In an evolutionary sense, IFN-γ developed early in the need for a more sophisticated immune response. IFN-γ *receptors* can be found on almost all cell types. This cytokine is the critical driver of a DTH response because of its ability to activate endothelial adhesion molecules and promote increased display of MHC class II markers on macrophages that promote maximal antigen presentation to Th1 cells.

In concert with its ability to amplify cellular inflammatory responses in general, INF-γ from antigen-activated Th1 cells also promotes antigen-specific B cell differentiation to plasma cells that produce phagocytosis-promoting IgG isotypes. The best tribute to the critical importance of IFN-γ to adequate antiviral DTH defenses is that viruses have encoded specific anti-IFN-γ strategies. Epstein-Barr virus, the virus that causes infectious mononucleosis and several lymphoproliferative diseases, hijacks the cytokine genes for IL-10. This provides Epstein-Barr virus with a cytokine-like action that strongly inhibits IFN-γ synthesis. Other viruses have evolved methods to produce soluble IFN-γ receptors that will blindfold the actual cytokine and inhibit its antiviral defenses.

The histologic appearance of a DTH reaction site is one of aggregated, activated, "angry" macrophages with lesser numbers of lymphocytes, neutrophils, and rare eosinophils. Depending on the vigor of the DTH response, macrophages can even fuse into the giant epithelioid cells, which produces the characteristic granulomatous appearance of many DTH reactions.

REGULATION OF DTH

The immune system must have counterregulatory strategies in place to dampen and finally turn off aggressive DTH responses. This crucial antagonist reaction is mobilized by activation of Th2 CD4 lymphocytes (Figure 13-2 and Table 13-2).

DTH can be a two-edged sword. Activated macrophages cause indiscriminate, innocent bystander tissue damage as they kill pathogens. If a DTH-promoting infection develops in vital organ sites, for example, tuberculosis in pulmonary tissue or certain viruses like Coxsackie virus in the endocrine portion of the pancreas, vital host tissue and organ functions can be lost during the cell-mediated response. It is not yet completely clear what factors are critical for initiating the shutdown of DTH, but several possibilities seem obvious. The successful suppression or eradication of an infection by DTH decreases or eliminates microbial antigen available for Th1 activation, and the genetically driven tempo and vigor of the immune response (possibly driven by the manner and efficiency of antigen presentation to the TCR) unique to the host are paramount. In any event, several

TABLE 13-2
T HELPER (Th) CELL CYTOKINE REGULATORY RELATIONSHIPS

CELL SOURCE	IL	PROMOTES SUBSET	INHIBITS SUBSET
M/M[1]	IL-12	Th1	–
M/M, NK, Th1	IFN-γ	Th1	Th2
Th2, basophil mast cell	IL-4	Th2	Th1
Th2, M/M	IL-10	Th2	Th1

[1]May also be made by other antigen-presenting cells.

critical changes in the cytokine milieu begin to occur as the intensity of DTH lessens. As microbial antigen load decreases, macrophage production of IL-12 decreases, and there is less promotion of Th1 differentiation. Simultaneously, in response to decreased IL-12 levels and further Th1 differentiation, IFN-γ levels decrease. The implications of decreased IFN-γ in the inflammatory site are significant. There is less macrophage activation, less endothelial display of adhesion ligands, and normalized display of MHC class II markers. *IL-4* released from mast cells, basophils, and previously activated Th2 cells now becomes the dominant cytokine. IL-4 is not only the primary driver of Th2 differentiation but also a strong antagonist to IFN-γ. *IL-10* production from both macrophages and the Th2 subset also increases. IL-10 is a key Th1 shutdown cytokine and the most potent antagonist of Th1 reactions. Once IL-10 prevails, there is usually dampening and ultimately shutdown of DTH. Histologically, fibrosis ensues, and the remaining intracellular pathogenic survivors are held in check by a delicate balance between antigen-specific, clonally expanded Th1 and Th2 CD4 subsets (Fig. 13-2).

DTH reactions can be exploited clinically for assessment of whether a patient has been infected previously with organisms that typically elicit DTH reactions. Common examples include tuberculosis, leprosy, many types of fungi, protozoans, and viruses. Key clinical data on whether the patient has been previously exposed to the organism and successfully mounted an antigen-specific DTH response can be gained by simply placing the antigen in question underneath the patient's epidermis and then assessing whether a micro-DTH response develops over the next 24 to 48 h (hence the derivation of the term DTH). Measurement of the inflammatory papule caused by the influx of macrophages and Th1 cells to the site of the antigen deposition confirms whether the patient has had a previous immunologic encounter with the organism and this information can be helpful in diagnosis and therapy. An additional benefit is that a positive DTH skin reaction suggests that the patient has general competence in Th1 host responses. Since effective promotion of DTH can exert a highly effective defense against an exposure to tuberculosis and leprosy, DTH can also be exploited for constructing vaccines to prevent diseases caused by DTH-evoking pathogens. The most common use of this strategy is to infect the patient with a live attenuated form of an organism to be protected against (e.g., BCG for tuberculosis). This method is successfully used in countries where tuberculous infection is rampant. A more contemporary strategy is to insert into vaccine preparations the genetic machinery for the production of cytokines that will drive a Th0 response to a Th1 response.

The need for a dynamic balance between Th subsets becomes evident when additional factors are superimposed on the host that can tilt the balance toward complete dominance of the Th2 subset or ineffective Th1 function. Suddenly, a few surviving intracellular pathogens, previously held in abeyance by macrophages and Th1 cells, thrive once again and threaten host survival. Destruction of an effective CD4 Th1 response by HIV or by the immunosuppressive therapy required in patients after organ transplantation are examples of acquired immunologic bankruptcy that leave the patient at risk for infection with usually innocuous organisms or reactivation of previously suppressed infections like tuberculosis. The implication of deficient DTH responses is evident in animal models. Genetic alteration of immune responses in mice that causes deficient Th1 responses (e.g., knock-out of IFN-γ or IL-12 genes) or an exogenous supply of IL-10 early after infection with DTH-inciting intracellular pathogens can lead to lack of containment by Th1 reactions and severe disseminated disease. Knock-out mice with no IFN-γ or IL-12 genes universally die after tuberculosis or Leishmania infection but survive if exogenous IFN-γ or IL-12 is provided at the time of infection. Conversely, the dark side of exuberant DTH reactions and severe tissue damage and organ failure becomes evident if the reactions are unchecked by the normal counterdynamics of IL-4 and IL-10 suppression. Finally, unraveling the intricacies of cytokine-effector cell communications that dictate the dominance of one subset over others will land ultimately to the ability to control and modulate cytokine expression. Therapeutic possibilities made feasible by this knowledge are limited only by the imagination. Already, genes for IL-12 production have been vectored into tumors to promote their own suicide by eliciting local intratumor DTH responses. Poorly controlled DTH autodirected (autoimmune) diseases such as rheumatoid arthritis and systemic lupus may be clinically modulated by up-regulating IL-10, and allergic diseases, like asthma, that are mediated by dominant Th2 responses to allergens may be suppressed by encouraging dominant Th1 responses.

COMPLEMENT VERSUS CELL-MEDIATED LYSIS

·

- **Complement**
    - **Classical Complement**
    - **Alternative Complement**
- **Cell-mediated Cytotoxicity**
    - **Necrosis**
    - **Apoptosis**

· · · · · · · · · · · ·

The immune system can kill cells via antibody utilizing the *complement* system or by *direct cell-mediated cytotoxicity*.

COMPLEMENT

Complement describes a group of approximately 20 heat-labile 24- to 550-kD normal serum proteins that together with antigen-bound antibodies act in an orderly sequence and in concert to produce various biological effects on cell membranes, one of which is lysis of cells or microorganisms. The complement system is the initiator of the inflammatory response and consists of two pathways: *classical* and *alternative*.

Classical complement

The classical complement pathway contains 11 different proenzyme proteins (C1-9) activated in sequence. C1 is the first component activated. C1 is composed of three subunits named C1q, C1r, and C1s. When a component is cleaved into a physiologic fragment(s), it is then designated by small letters (e.g., C3a, C3b).

When a single complement enzyme or complex is active, it is so designated with a bar over the active component (e.g., active C4 is C$\overline{4}$).

It should be realized that the C components (Table 14-1) were named in the order of their discovery before their function was known; thus, their names do not

TABLE 14-1
COMPLEMENT COMPONENTS

PROTEIN		FUNCTION
NATIVE	**ACTIVE**	
Classical Pathway		
C1 Complex		
	C1q	Binds Fc region of IgM, IgG1, 3, 2($\pm$)
	C1r	Serum protease: enzymatically activates C1s
	C1s	Serum protease: cleaves C4 which cleaves C2
C4	C4a	Weak peptide mediator of inflammation (anaphyla-toxin)
	C4b	Binds C2 for cleavage by C1s—C$\overline{4b2a}$
C2	C2a	Serine protease: C$\overline{4b2a}$ (C3 convertase)
	C2b	Kinin
C3	C3a	Intermediate peptide mediator of inflammation (anaphylatoxin)
	C3b	Forms C5 convertase with C$\overline{4b2a}$; Opsonin: Initi-ates alternate pathway amplification
Alternative Pathway		
C3	C3b	Binds B for cleavage by D
Factor B		
	Ba	Unknown function
	Bb	Serine protease: Active enzyme of C$\overline{3bBb}$ (C3 con-vertase) which generates C3bBb3b (C5 convertase)
D	D	Serine protease: Cleaves B bound to C3b forming Ba and Bb
Properdin	Properdin	Stabilizes C$\overline{3bBb}$
Terminal		
(Both Pathways)		
C5	C5a	Small peptide mediator of inflammation (anaphyla-toxin); Chemotaxis
	C5b	Binds C6 to form nucleus of MAC
C6	C6	C$\overline{5b6}$ binds C7
C7	C7	C$\overline{5b67}$ binds C8; amphiphilic transition inserts into lipid bilayer
C8	C8	C$\overline{5b678}$ binds 10-16 C9 molecules initiating its polymerization
C9	C9	Polymerizes to C$\overline{5b678}$ to form a MAC

(continued)

TABLE 14-1
(CONTINUED)

PROTEIN		FUNCTION
NATIVE	**ACTIVE**	
Regulatory Proteins	**Pathway Affected**	
Soluble		
C1 inhibitor	Classical (Cla)	Binds $C1\overline{rs}$ removing it from $C\overline{1q}$
C4b-binding protein	Cla	Binds to $C\overline{4b}$ displacing $C\overline{2a}$; cofactor for C4b cleavage by I
Factor H	Alternate (A)	
		Binds $C\overline{3b}$ displacing $\overline{Bb}$; I cofactor
Factor I		
(C3b Inactivator)	Cla and A	Serine protease which cleaves $C\overline{4b}$ or $C\overline{3b}$ using H, DAF, MCP, C4bBp or CR1 as cofactors
S Protein	Terminal	Binds C5b67 and prevents membrane insertion
Membrane Bound		
Complement Receptor 1		
(CR1)	Cla and A	Promotes C4b and C3b inactivation by factor I
Membrane Cofactor		
Protein (MCP)		
Decay-accelerating	Cla and A	Displaces C2b from C4b and Bb from C3b
factor (DAF)		
Homologous Restriction		
Factor		
(HRF)	Terminal	Binds $C\overline{5b678}$ blocking C9 binding and preventing MAC formation
CD59 (protectin)	Terminal	Binds $C\overline{5b678}$ blocking C9 binding and preventing MAC formation

Receptors	**Ligands**	**Cells**	**Functions**
CR1 (CD35)	C3b, C4b	Erythrocytes (E),	E transport of immune complexes;
		Phagocytic Cells,	Stimulates phagocytosis;
		FDC, B Cells	Promotes C3b and C4b decay
CR2 (CD21)	C3b inactive (i);	B Cells,	Part of B cell coreceptor;
	Epstein-Barr (EB) virus	FDC	Binds E-B virus
CR3 (CD11b/18)	C3bi	Phagocytic Cells	Binding then phagocytosis of immune complexes;
		FDC	Facilitation of neutrophil
CR4 (CD11c/18)	C3bi	Phagocytic Cells	Extravasation by cell-adhesion molecule binding.

reflect their reaction sequence. The classical pathway is initiated after the C1 complex binds to an Ag-Ab complex deposited on a cell surface. This recognition is possible because Ag binding to IgG1, IgG2, IgG3, or IgM exposes a binding site on the C_H2 domain of the antibody's F_c portion (Fig. 14-1). C1 in serum is a 750-kD macromolecular Ca^{2+}-dependent complex consisting of a C1q and two molecules each of C1r and C1s ($C1qr_2s_2$). C1q consists of 18 polypeptide chains, which form six collagen-like triple-helical arms with a globular head similar to a bunch of six tulips. When the tips of the C1q tulip bind the C_H2 domain of two IgG molecules within 30 to 40 nm of each other or bind only one molecule of IgM, they activate the enzymatic activity in $C1r_2$. Active $C1r_2$ cleaves and activates the associated serine protease $C1s_2$; thus, an active C1 ($C1qr_2s_2$) is produced. The $C1s_2$ splits C4 into two fragments, C4a and C4b. C4b covalently binds to cell surface antigen and in the presence of Mg^{2+} binds and activates C2, generating C2a and C2b. C2 can also be activated by C1s to generate C2a and C2b. C2b acts as a kinin and increases vascular permeability, causing swelling, edema, and pain. C2a then joins the C4b on the cell surface, forming C4b2a (convertase), which acts as a powerful C3 convertase as it splits numerous C3 molecules into C3b and C3a, thus causing pathway amplification.

C3a is an anaphylatoxin that causes mast cell degranulation, smooth muscle contraction, and increased capillary permeability. C3b binds to a nearby membrane component and joins C42 on the cell surface, forming a new enzyme complex, C423, which can cleave many C5 peptides into C5a and C5b. C5a also acts as an anaphylatoxin as well as a chemotactic factor attracting leukocytes to an inflammatory site. The unstable C5b joins one molecule of C6, forming the stable C56 complex; this complex binds in turn one molecule of C7, leading to formation of the C567, which inserts into the lipid bilayers of cell membranes. C8 can join this complex, forming C5678. The C5678 is responsible for slow membrane leakage. However, C5678 can subsequently bind up to six molecules of C9, forming a trans-membrane channel, which can result in cellular osmotic leakage. This C5b6789 complex is thus called the membrane attack complex (MAC).

Alternative complement

The alternative complement pathway is antibody-independent but dependent on the ability of certain microbial surface antigens to activate C3. Factor B (similar to C2), factor D (active serine protease similar to $C1qr_2s_2$) and properdin play important roles in the alternative pathway.

The pathway begins with the hydrolysis of C3 into C3a and C3b by microbial products such as lipopolysaccharide. C3b binds to microorganism cell membranes, and in the presence of Mg^{2+}, it binds serum factor B, which is a substrate for active factor D. Factor D is a plasma serine proteinase and circulates in the blood in an active form. Factor D cleaves B, releasing Ba and generating C3bBb, which acts as a C3 convertase similar to C4b2a of the classical pathway. Pro-

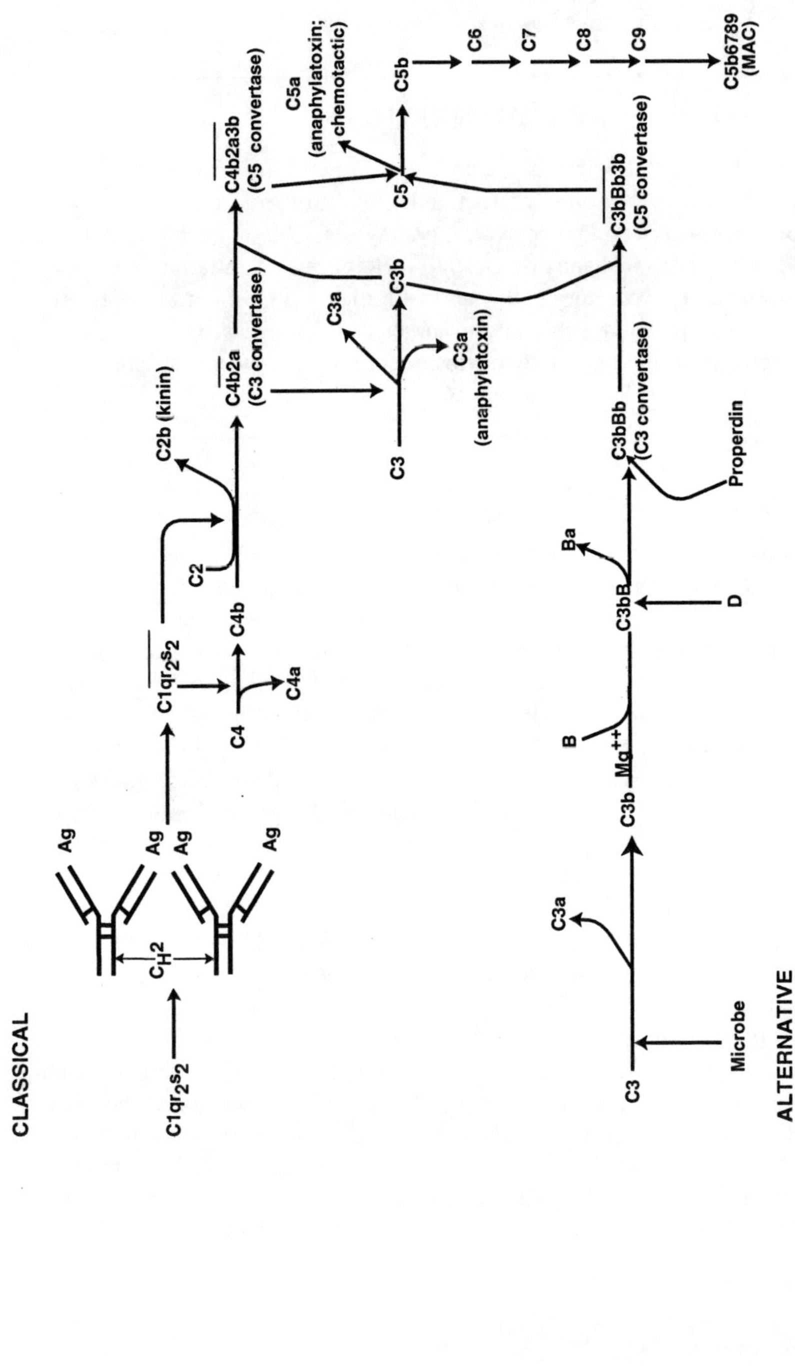

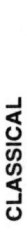

CLASSICAL

ALTERNATIVE

Figure 14-1
Complement pathways.

perdin binds to $\overline{\text{C3bBb}}$, stabilizing it and allowing it to activate more unhydrolyzed C3, thus amplifying the process and producing many C3bBb3b complexes on the cell surface. This complex acts as C5 convertase, since it binds C5 and hydrolyzes it to C5a (chemotactic) and C5b. C5b then initiates formation of the membrane attack complex as in the classical pathway.

CELL-MEDIATED CYTOTOXICITY

Cell-mediated cytotoxicity is the ability of armed effector cells to recognize some receptor(s) on the target cells, bind to them, and initiate their demise by either secretory (perforin, granzymes, TNFα) or non-secretory (Fas/Fas ligand) mechanisms. Despite differences in initiation, both the secretory and nonsecretory pathways can initiate very similar downstream events that eventually culminate in target cell *apoptosis*. However, it is only perforin in the granule exocytosis secretory pathway that can cause *lysis* of target cells leading to *necrosis*.

Necrosis

There are specific and nonspecific cytotoxic cells. Specific cytotoxic cells are mostly $CD8^+$ (a few are $CD4^+$) that recognize their target cell that is presenting a 6- to 9-amino acid cognate peptide via its major histocompatibility complex (MHC) class I molecule. Such MHC-restricted recognition causes the $CD8^+$ cell to either exocytose granules containing perforin and granzymes (A and B) or to secrete cytotoxic cytokines such as TNFα/β. When the monomeric protein perforin is released in the presence of Ca^{2+}, there is enzymic polymerization of the perforin, forming polyperforin channels on the target cell similar to those formed by the C9 component of complement system. If enough of these channels are formed, the cell will undergo lysis contributing to necrosis. Granzymes, also present in the $CD8^+$ cell granules, are released into the target cell through polyperforin channels. If perforin does not cause lysis, these serine proteases can take part in the apoptotic pathway by activating caspase 3. $CD8^+$ cells can also secrete TNFα/β, which, upon binding to the TNF receptor type 1 (p55) (TNFR1), can also activate caspase 8 and the subsequent caspase cascade (Fig. 14-2).

Nonspecific cytotoxicity is mainly carried out by natural killer (NK) cells, but macrophages may also contribute; however, there may be a specific component to their initial activation. While the CD3/TCR receptor complexes on $CD8^+$ T cells look for self MHC I and non-self peptide in order to function, $CD3^-/TCR^-CD16^+CD56^+$ NK cells look for lack of self MHC I on target cells. Since some tumor cells and viral infected cells do not express, or express low levels of cell surface MHC I, these cells are susceptible to NK-mediated killing. NK

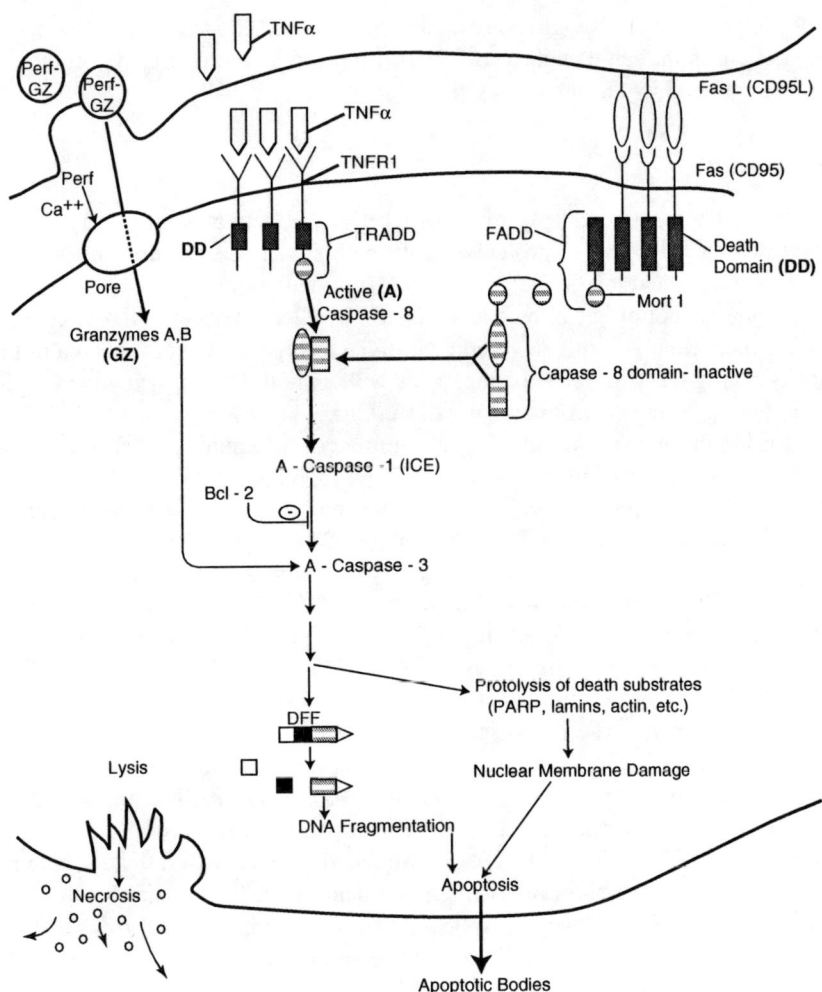

Figure 14-2
Cell-mediated cytotoxicity: CD8$^+$ cytotoxic T cell.

cell killing can be enhanced by interleukin-2 (IL-2). When NK cells are incubated *in vitro* with IL-2 for 1 to 2 days, these activated cells are then called lympho-kine-activated killer (LAK) cells. Also, NK and LAK cells as well as macro-phages can also kill target cells coated with noncomplement-fixing antibodies by binding to the F_c piece of the antibody via their F_c receptor. Once their F_c recep-tor is activated, they release perforin/granzyme granules similar to CD8$^+$ T cells. This method of killing is called antibody-dependent cell-mediated cytotoxicity, or ADCC. However, it should be realized that NK-, LAK-, and ADCC-mediated killing occur in the same manner as CTL, with perforin and granzyme containing granules released by all three cell types.

Apoptosis

Apoptosis is a form of cell death in which the cell activates an internal lethal enzyme cascade leading to proteolysis of death substrates, membrane changes, nuclear damage, and internucleosome DNA fragmentation.

Apoptosis not only can be caused by CTL, NK, LAK, and ADCC cells; it also occurs normally during development of T cells in the subcortical area of the thymus among $CD4^+8^+$ cells (Chap. 5) as well as in the basal light zone of germinal centers during centrocyte maturation (Chap. 11).

It is important to realize that while a number of different external stimuli and molecules can activate apoptotic mechanisms in other cells, only FAS ligand (FAS-L)/FAS (CD95L/CD95), TNFα/TNFR1, and perforin/granzyme B granule exocytosis are activated after T cell receptor (TCR) engagement of foreign peptide-MHC on target cells. After TCR engagement, signals are transduced into the T cell to activate transcription and expression of the homotrimer FAS-L on its surface (Fig. 14-3). FAS-L binds to target cells expressing FAS in a Ca^{2+}-independent manner, inducing the trimerization of FAS and activating a sequence of events that leads to downstream activation of the caspase system, leading to apoptosis of target cells. The cytoplasmic tail of FAS contains a unique 80-amino acid sequence, which is conserved among receptor-mediated apoptic pathways and is thus referred to as the death domain (DD). When FAS engages FAS-L, DDs are activated and trimerized, leading to recruitment of several intracellular proteins. One of these is FADD (FAS-associated protein with a death domain), which has a DD at the N-terminal end and a death effector domain (MORT1) at the C-terminal end. MORT1 is responsible for downstream signal transduction. Caspase-8, which has two death-effector domains, is the next protein to be recruited to this complex via MORT/MORT interaction. When appropriate FAS/FAS-L interaction occurs with consequent FADD/MORT1 activation, there is a cleavage of caspase-8 proenzyme. Active caspase-8 is then formed, which activates caspase-1 and then caspase-3. Caspase-3 then cleaves a number of nuclear and cytoplasmic proenzymes. One group of proenzymes that caspase-3 causes proteolysis of is a group of death substrates (poly ADP-ribose poly-merases (PARPS), lamins, actin) that cause morphological changes in the nuclear membrane. Another proenzyme is DNA fragmentation factor, which caspase-3 cleaves into three fragments, one of which causes DNA fragmentation.

Caspase-8, -1, and -3 referred to above are just three in a series of specific cellular serine proteases important in execution of the apoptotic pathway. All cas-pases share three key features: they all have cysteine at their active site, they require an aspartic acid at the cleavage site, and they are all synthesized as proen-zymes that are activated by cleavage at aspartate residues at sites resembling their own targets. Thus, some transactivation and consequent autoprocessing among caspases can occur. Also, as mentioned above, the serine protease granzyme B released from granules can also activate caspase-3. In addition, the release of TNFα from a cytotoxic cell that binds to the TNFR1 on the target activates a TRADD (TNF receptor-associated protein with a death domain), which can also activate caspase-8. Finally, it should be appreciated that a protein found in high concentration on the outer mitochondrial membrane, Bcl-2 (B cell leukemia fac-tor 2) blocks the caspase pathway at the caspase-1 level, not allowing active cas-pase-3 to form.

Thus, cytotoxic cells can kill targets in two ways: necrosis and apoptosis. *Necrosis* is mainly caused by a high concentration of 70-kD glycoprotein perforin monomers, which in the presence of Ca^{2+} insert themselves into target cell mem-brane similar to C9 and subsequently aggregate to form homopolymeric 5- to 20-nm pore structures. Thus, water and low molecular weight solutes freely enter tar-get cells, causing colloid-osmotic lysis or bursting of cells leading to cell lysis and possibly necrosis. *Apoptosis* can be caused by FAS/FAS-L, TNFα/TNFR1, or granzyme B activation of the caspase system cascade, which leads to mem-brane damage and DNA fragmentation. The result is membrane-bound cell cleavage products called apoptotic bodies, which are easily phagocytosed by sur-rounding macrophages with no tissue necrosis. However, unlike perforin, which causes irreversible cell lysis similar to the final products of the complement cas-cade, the cell surface signals that activate the caspase cascade can be blocked by the mitochondrial protein Bcl-2. Thus, there is an internal brake for apoptosis.

Recent studies in tumor immunology indicate that some tumor cells can actually produce FAS-L, which can complex with FAS on some potential effec-tor T cells, thus eliminating them. Thus, the opposite of Fig. 14-3 is produced.

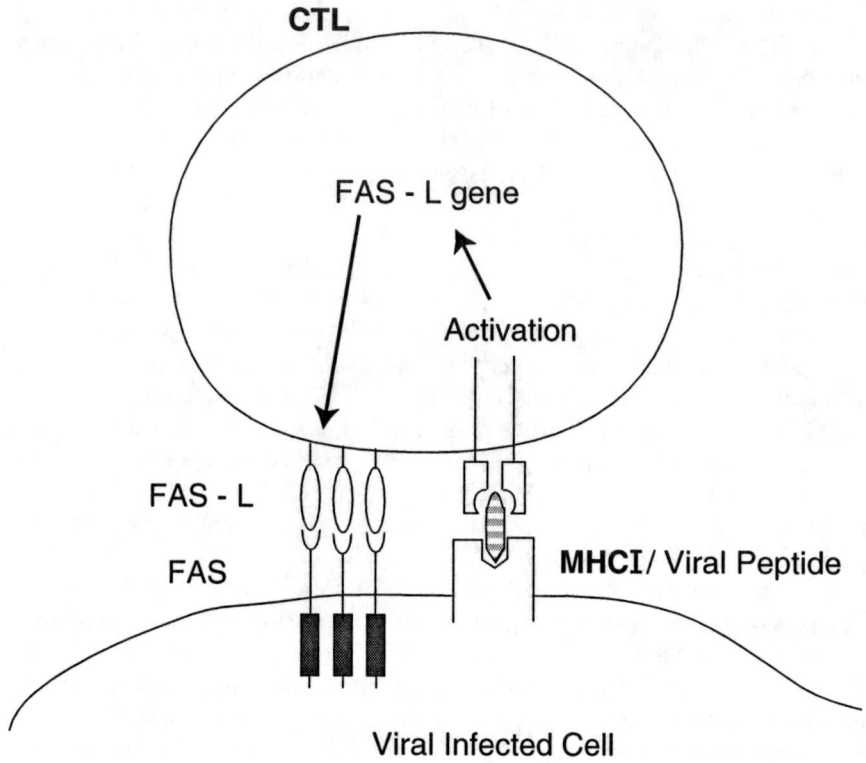

Figure 14-3
Induction of FAS-L.

MICROBIAL IMMUNITY AND IMMUNOPARASITOLOGY

·

- **Nonspecific (Innate) Immunity**
- **Specific (Adaptive) Immunity**

  Bacterial Infection

  Viral Infection

  Parasitic Infection

· · · · · · · · · · · · ·

NONSPECIFIC (INNATE) IMMUNITY

Nonspecific immunity refers to mechanisms of protection that do not require specific recognition of antigen, but that increase the protection afforded by specific immune mechanisms. Nonspecific immune mechanisms include phagocytosis, acute inflammatory responses, type I interferons, and tumor necrosis factor (see Chap. 1).

Our ability to combat the many microorganisms that gain entry into our bodies daily depends on both nonspecific and specific mechanisms. Some nonspecific mechanisms include those that either kill or prevent the spread of microorganisms at their point of entry into the host. For example, bacteria are either killed on the skin by the low pH conditions that are created on the skin by the release of lactic acid in sweat gland secretions or are killed by mucous secretions, such as tears and saliva, that contain lysozyme, an enzyme that disrupts the cell wall of Gram-positive bacteria to cause their death.

Once the microorganism gains entry into the body, other nonspecific mechanisms take over. *Phagocytosis* is a mechanism used by neutrophils and macrophages to engulf microorganisms that adhere to their surface and then degrade them in intracellular lysosomal compartments. Within the cell, the engulfed microorganism is destroyed by superoxide anions, hydrogen peroxide, or the low pH environment of a lysosomal compartment that contains numerous enzymes to degrade the microorganism. Some individuals are especially vulnerable to chronic infections, such as patients with chronic granulomatous disease, because they have phagocytic cells that cannot produce superoxide anions. In addition, the entry of microorganisms into the body induces an *acute inflammatory response* against the microorganisms that involves the production of a number of plasma proteins to help combat the infection. These plasma proteins include C-reactive protein and complement, both of which nonspecifically coat bacteria to enhance their phagocytosis by neutrophils and macrophages.

A number of cytokines also provide a nonspecific mechanism to control the expansion of invading microorganisms in the body. *Type I interferons (IFNs)*, IFN-α and IFN-β, are produced by macrophages and fibroblasts, respectively, in response to viral infections (see Appendix 2). Type I interferons inhibit viral replication, increase MHC class I expression, and decrease MHC class II expression, thus preferentially slanting the immune response toward a CD8+ cell-mediated response (see Chap. 7), and increase natural killer cell activity to kill virally-infected cells. Also, *tumor necrosis factor α (TNFα)* is produced by endotoxin (active component of Gram-negative bacteria)-activated macrophages to induce neutrophils to adhere to the vascular endothelium. This attachment of neutrophils to the vascular endothelium increases the number of cells that accumulate at the site of inflammation and, thus, increases the synthesis of plasma proteins by the neutrophils that are associated with the acute inflammatory response. Interleukin (IL)-1 is another cytokine that controls the expansion of microorganisms in the body by its ability to induce fever and, in a manner similar to TNFα, increases the synthesis of plasma proteins by the neutrophils and macrophages that are associated with the acute inflammatory response.

SPECIFIC (ADAPTIVE) IMMUNITY

Specific immunity consists of mechanisms of protection that require specific recognition of antigen. Specific immune mechanisms include the processes involved in humoral and cell-mediated immunity (see Chap. 1).

Bacterial infection

• **ROLE OF HUMORAL IMMUNITY**   The most efficient mechanism for eliminating extracellular bacteria from the host is through phagocytosis. This is a process by which phagocytic cells such as macrophages, monocytes, and neutrophils engulf bacteria that adhere to their surface and then degrade them in intracellular lysosomal compartments. However, a number of deadly organisms, such as encapsulated pneumococci, do not nonspecifically adhere well to phagocytic cells.

Specific immune mechanisms need to be used to promote the adherence of extracellular bacteria to phagocytic cells. These mechanisms involve the production of IgM and IgG antibodies and the activation of complement.

The cell wall and capsule of most bacteria are polysaccharides and, thus, act as T cell-independent antigens for antibody production (discussed in Chap. 9). This particular mechanism for inducing antibody production is good for the host because it provides means by which bacteria can directly activate B cells to produce IgM antibody. In addition, it is possible to induce IgG antibody production through this mechanism, but only when T cell-derived cytokines, such as IL-4 and IFN-γ, are present. These cytokines are produced by T cells that have been activated through either exposure to a superantigen or interaction with APCs presenting processed bacterial antigen in association with class II MHC (discussed in Chap. 7). As depicted in Fig. 15-1, the IgM and IgG antibodies bind to either cell surface bacterial antigens or secreted bacterial toxins, thus, activating the C3 components of complement. It is then the complement component that binds to complement receptors on phagocytic cells to promote the phagocytosis of the antibody-coated bacteria or toxin. In addition, IgG antibodies that bind to both cell surface bacterial antigens and secreted toxins bind to special receptors on phagocytic cells that bind to the Fc portion of IgG antibodies called *Fcγ receptors*. The binding of antigen-bound IgG to Fcγ receptors also promotes efficient phagocytosis. This mechanism of specific immunity applies to persons receiving tetanus toxin vaccine. In these cases, the toxin released by the tetanus bacteria is bound by the IgG that has been produced against it. The tetanus toxin-IgG complex then binds to phagocytes via the Fcγ receptor and promotes the destruction of the toxin.

• ROLE OF CELL-MEDIATED IMMUNITY

IFN-γ plays a critical role in protection against intracellular bacteria. The activation of macrophages by IFN-γ produced by T cells is the critical stage of protection against intracellular bacterial organisms. In this manner, IFN-γ stimulates many macrophages to phagocytose and destroy the microorganism.

Some bacteria, including *Listeria monocytogenes*, *Mycobacterium tuberculosis*, and *Mycobacterium leprae*, are engulfed by phagocytes but are essentially resistant to degradation by lysosomal enzymes due to the lack of fusion between lysosomal vesicles and the vesicles in which the microorganisms grow. As a consequence, these organisms survive within the cell and, therefore, cannot be recognized by any antibody that may be circulating in the serum. Instead, cell-mediated immune mechanisms are activated to protect the host. Although these

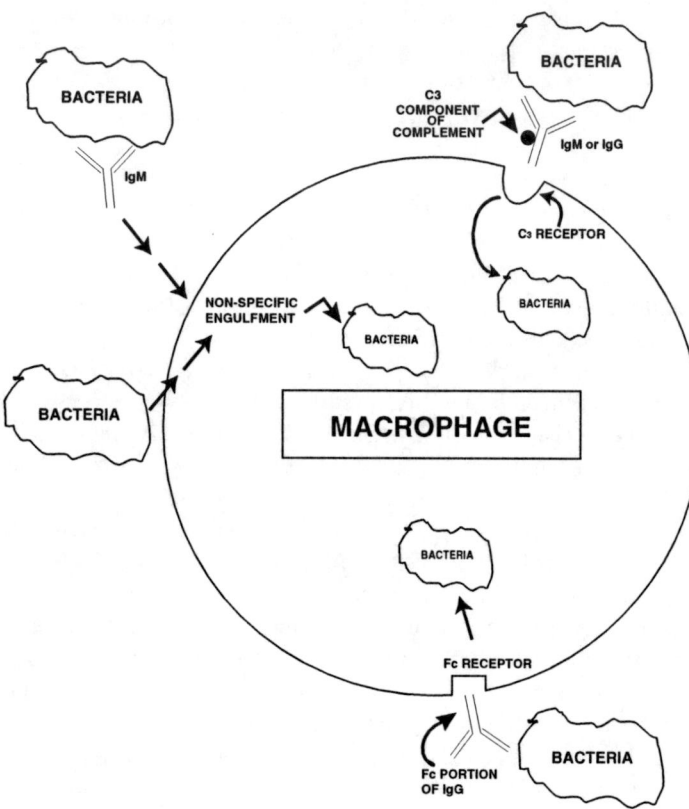

Figure 15-1
Humoral mechanisms of specific immunity against bacteria.

microorganisms are essentially resistant to lysosomal enzymes within macrophages, a few macrophages do become activated, inducing the fusion between lysosomal vesicles and vesicles containing the microorganism and allowing for the production of peptide fragments that can effectively associate with MHC class I and II. The T cells involved in the cell-mediated immune response include the CD8+ and CD4+ T cells that become activated upon T cell receptor recognition of bacterial antigens presented by macrophages in association with MHC class I or class II molecules, respectively. T cell activation induces the production of IFN-γ, which, in turn, leads to the further activation of macrophages, including those macrophages that are not infected.

This mechanism for developing immunity against one particular intracellular organism explains why the host not only is immune to subsequent challenge

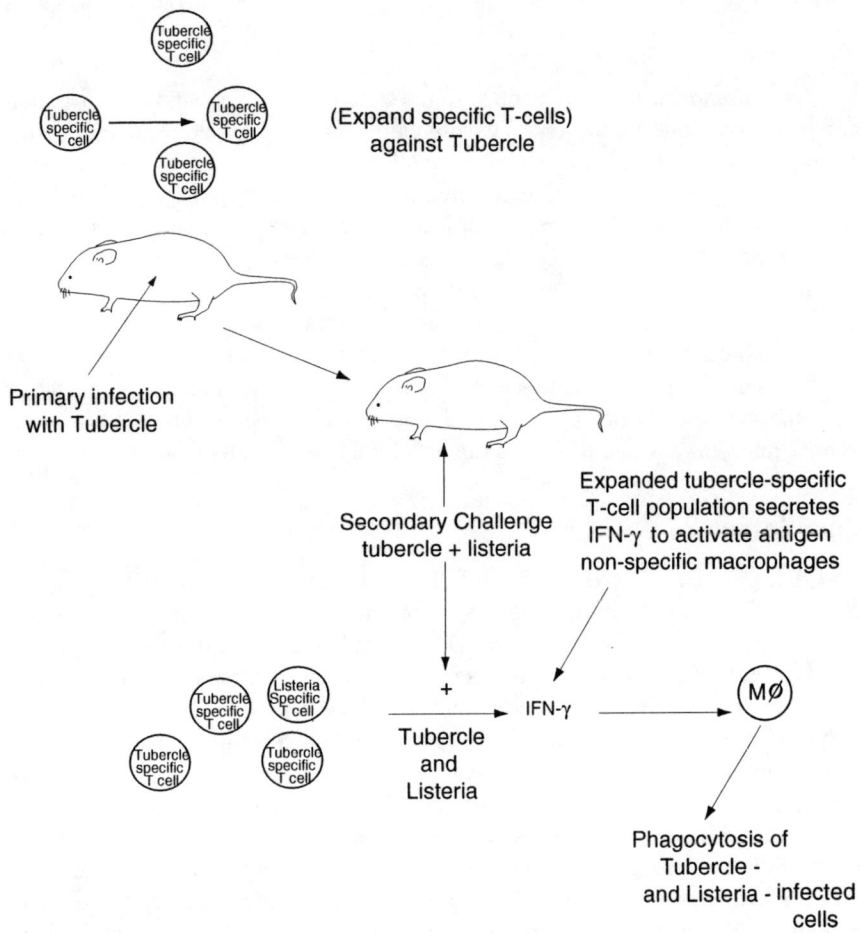

Figure 15-2
Specific immune reactions can induce nonspecific immune mechanisms.

with the original intracellular organism but also is immune to subsequent challenge with other intracellular microorganisms given at the same time. As shown in Fig. 15-2, the original microorganism (e.g., mycobacterium tuberculosis which produces a tubercle) stimulates the expansion of the few tubercle-specific T cells that may be present in the host. Upon subsequent exposure to tubercle and another unrelated microorganism, the expanded population of tubercle-specific T cells becomes activated to secrete IFN-γ, which, in turn, acts on macrophages to activate phagocytosis. Since macrophage functions are antigen-nonspecific, any microorganism within the environment of an activated macrophage will be effectively eliminated. Therefore, the specificity of this immune response lies in the activation of the expanded clone of T cells specific for recognition of the original organism.

Granulomas result from a collection of activated macrophages that accumulate in an area due to the chronic antigenic stimulation that results from the chronic presence of highly resistant intracellular bacteria.

One clinical outcome from cell-mediated immune responses against intracellular bacteria is the development of granulomas. The presence of these granulomas is diagnostic of chronic mycobacterial infections.

It is also clear that CD4+ subsets may be differentially involved in cell-mediated immune responses against different types of leprosy. In lepromatous leprosy, which is characterized by a marked accumulation of an intracellular microorganism, IL-4 production by CD4+ T cells is dominant. On the other hand, in tuberculoid leprosy, which is characterized by the presence of few intracellular microorganisms, IFN-γ production by CD4+ T cells is dominant.

Viral infection

• **ROLE OF HUMORAL IMMUNITY**   A virus enters a host cell by binding to molecules that are normally expressed on the host cell surface for use in normal cell functions. For example, the CD4 molecule on T cells is a critical cell surface molecule that is used for the recognition of antigen presented by an APC (described in detail in Chap. 7). However, the HIV-1 gains entry into a host cell by binding to the CD4 molecule expressed by T-helper lymphocytes. Therefore, it is essential that a mechanism exist to neutralize and clear the virus before it attaches to a host cell surface molecule. This mechanism involves antibody directed against the virus. The specific antibodies can either bind to the virus site that binds to the host cell surface molecule to prevent its attachment or bind to the virus and enhance the probability of the virus being phagocytosed and destroyed, or they can activate complement that will either enhance phagocytosis or direct lysis of the virus.

Antibody-mediated immunity against viruses is effective primarily during the early stages of a viral infection before virus entry into the host cell. Since antibodies are unable to penetrate cells to bind to intracellular microorganisms, their effectiveness is limited to the times when the virus is outside the cell, which is during either early infection or viral release from the host cell. Also, it is difficult to establish long-term protection against a virus, since the surface antigenic structure of the virus can change to create a different viral strain. This is particularly relevant in the case of the common cold, which is caused by a rhinovirus that is usually serotypically distinct during each infection. However, secretory IgA may offer some protection at the sites of rhinovirus entry, namely the nose and lungs.

• **ROLE OF CELL-MEDIATED IMMUNITY**   The most important cellular mechanism for protection against viruses is provided for by the CD8+ T lymphocyte. The CD8+ T cell recognizes viral antigens that have been processed and

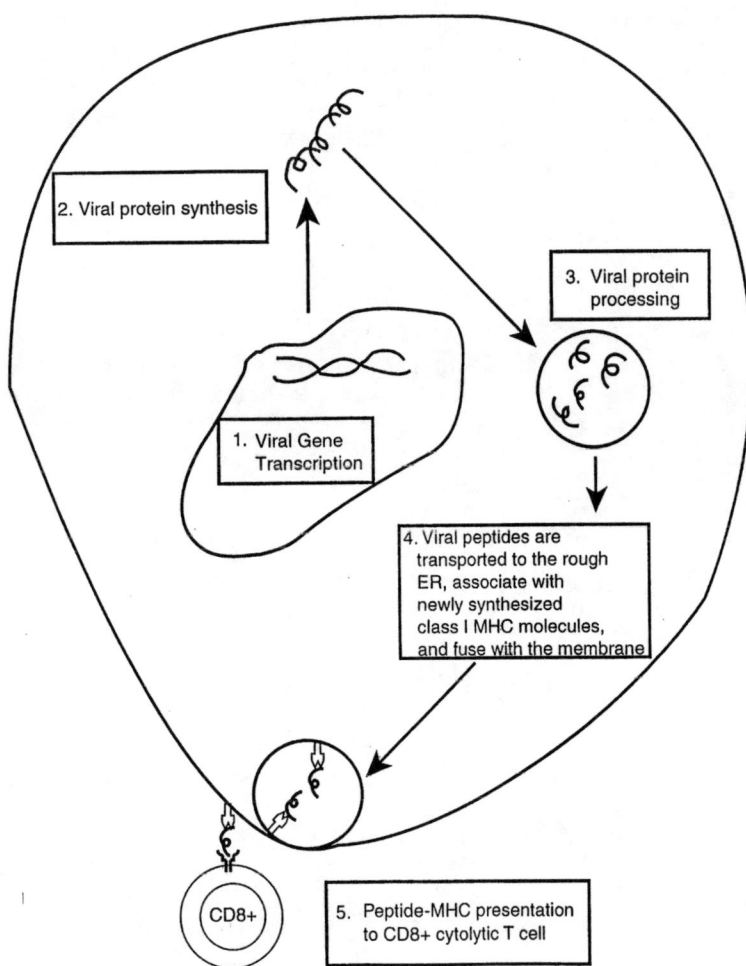

2. Viral protein synthesis

3. Viral protein processing

1. Viral Gene Transcription

4. Viral peptides are transported to the rough ER, associate with newly synthesized class I MHC molecules, and fuse with the membrane

CD8+

5. Peptide-MHC presentation to CD8+ cytolytic T cell

Figure 15-3 Virus-infected cell.
Pathway of class I MHC-restricted presentation of an endogenously synthesized viral antigen.

associated with MHC class I molecules for expression on the cell surface (Fig. 15-3). The complex of viral antigen and MHC class I on the cell surface is recognized by receptors on specific CD8+ T cells. To fully differentiate into cytolytic T cells, the CD8+ T cell requires cytokine "help" from CD4+ T cells that are activated by viral antigen in association with MHC class II molecules on the surface of specialized antigen-presenting cells, such as macrophages, that

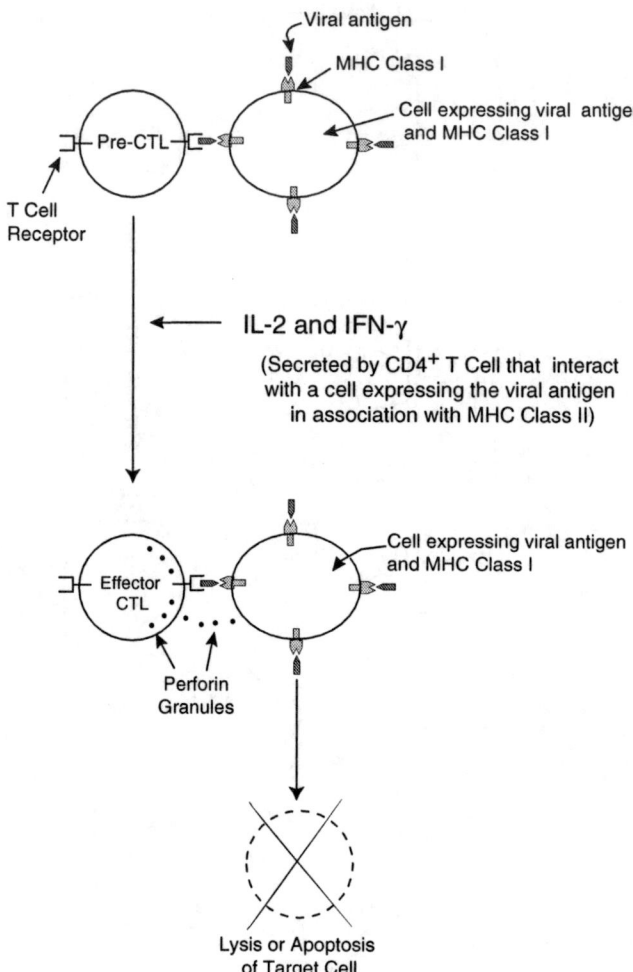

Figure 15-4
Cytokines allow for the differentiation of CD8+ cytolytic T cells into effector cells.

have phagocytized antibody-coated extracellular virus (Fig. 15-4). The cytokine "help" provided by CD4+ T cells, which includes the cytokines IL-2 and IFN-γ, induces the differentiation and expansion of virus-specific CD8+ T cells. Therefore, the ability of CD8+ T cells to lyse and destroy a virally infected cell is critically dependent on the early action of cytokines derived from CD4+ T cells. The mechanism of cell-mediated immune protection against viral infections is a good example of how concurrent class I- and class II-mediated T cell activation of CD8+ and CD4+ T cells, respectively, works to protect the host against viruses.

Parasitic infection

• **ROLE OF HUMORAL IMMUNITY** Parasites include the helminths, such as schistisomes, and protozoa, such as the malaria organism *Plasmodium*. Parasites are infectious organisms that go through part of their life cycle in the human host and part of their life cycle in an intermediate host, such as a fly, tick, snail, or mosquito. For example, malaria is transmitted to humans from mosquito bites, while schistosomiasis is transmitted by the water from areas in which reside infected snails.

A major mechanism of defense against parasites is the production of IgE. The production of IgE is very much dependent on the production of IL-4 by CD4+ Th2 cells (discussed in more detail in Chap. 13). As a consequence of the action of IL-4 on parasite-activated B cells, parasite-specific IgE antibodies are produced that opsonize the parasitic organism. The opsonized parasite then binds to eosinophils through the Fc portion of the IgE to induce the release of proteins that lyse the parasite. Eosinophils are primarily involved in this type of protection because parasites seem to be more susceptible to destruction by toxic proteins released by eosinophils as compared with the toxic proteins and reactive oxygen species released by macrophages and neutrophils.

Persistent parasite infections lead to the formation of many parasite-antibody complexes that not only attach to eosinophils but also attach to blood vessels and the glomerulus of the kidney. The latter attachments produce detrimental consequences, such as the development of vasculitis and nephritis. These are major complications in persons with malaria.

• **ROLE OF CELL-MEDIATED IMMUNITY** As described above for viruses, the most important cellular mechanism for protection against parasites is the CD8+ T lymphocyte. The CD8+ T cell recognizes endogenously produced parasite antigens that have been processed and associated with MHC class I molecules. The complex of parasite antigen and MHC class I is recognized by specific T cells expressing the T cell receptor and CD8. Also, as discussed above, the CD4+ T cell is intimately involved in effective CD8+ T cell function by providing cytokines needed for CD8+ T cell differentiation and expansion.

However, parasites are very clever microorganisms when it comes to evading immune defense mechanisms. Two of the more important evasion strategies used by parasites include 1) the ability of parasites to acquire an outer coat of host proteins so that these proteins, as opposed to the parasite outer membrane proteins, will not be recognized as antigens and, therefore, not attach antigen-specific IgE; and 2) the ability of parasites to shed their cell surface membranes after specific IgE antibodies have attached in order to prevent IgE-mediated attachment of the parasite to eosinophils.

AUTOIMMUNITY

•

- **B Cell Tolerance**
- **Clonal Deletion**
- **Clonal Anergy**
- **Immunogen vs. Tolerogen**
- **B Cell-associated Autoimmune Diseases**
- **Mechanisms for Breaking B Cell Tolerance**
- **Molecular Mimicry**
- **Polyclonal B Cell Activation**
- **Polyclonal T Cell Activation**
- **Superantigens**
- **Exposure of "Hidden" Self Antigens**

•   •   •   •   •   •   •   •   •   •   •   •

A basic premise of the B cell response to antigen is that the B cell will secrete antibodies against anything that is not normally present in the body. These antibodies will eliminate the antigen before it causes damage to the host. The B cell recognizes antigens via the immunoglobulin receptor that is expressed on its cell surface. As discussed in Chap. 4, the immunoglobulin receptor is formed by a series of gene deletions and recombinations during the process of B cell maturation in the bone marrow. Therefore, millions of different immunoglobulin variable regions are produced during B cell maturation. This results in the production of millions of B cells that are able to recognize millions of different antigens, including those "antigens" that normally do exist in the body.

Unlike T cell maturation and selection in the thymus, no well characterized mechanism exists in the bone marrow to delete B cells that recognize molecules that normally exist in the body. If left unchecked, B cells would produce antibodies against all of the proteins in the body. This situation would lead to massive destruction of cells through either cell destruction by antibody/complement-mediated cell lysis mechanisms or the removal of critical protein molecules, such as serum albumin, by antibody-dependent elimination mechanisms. Needless to say, this does not normally occur. Therefore, some mechanism must exist that makes B cells unresponsive to antigens normally considered "self." This mechanism is called *tolerance*.

B CELL TOLERANCE

B cell tolerance is a process that involves the failure of a B cell to respond to foreign or self antigen.

There are two basic mechanisms of B cell tolerance. One mechanism involves the elimination of reactive B cells through the process of clonal deletion. The other mechanism involves the process of clonal anergy.

CLONAL DELETION

This process involves the elimination of immature B cells after antigen binds to their immunoglobulin receptor.

An immature B cell that is just leaving the bone marrow expresses predominantly IgM on its surface. This is in contrast to a mature B cell, which expresses both IgM and IgD on its surface. It seems that when antigen binds to IgM only, a lethal signal is delivered to the B cell (Fig. 16-1). This is in contrast to the stimulatory signal that is delivered to the B cell if antigen binds to both IgM and IgD. However, this mechanism of B cell tolerance is not well supported by scientific data and, therefore, probably does not represent the major mechanism of B cell tolerance.

CLONAL ANERGY

This process involves the inability of mature B cells to respond to antigen even after it binds to its immunoglobulin receptor.

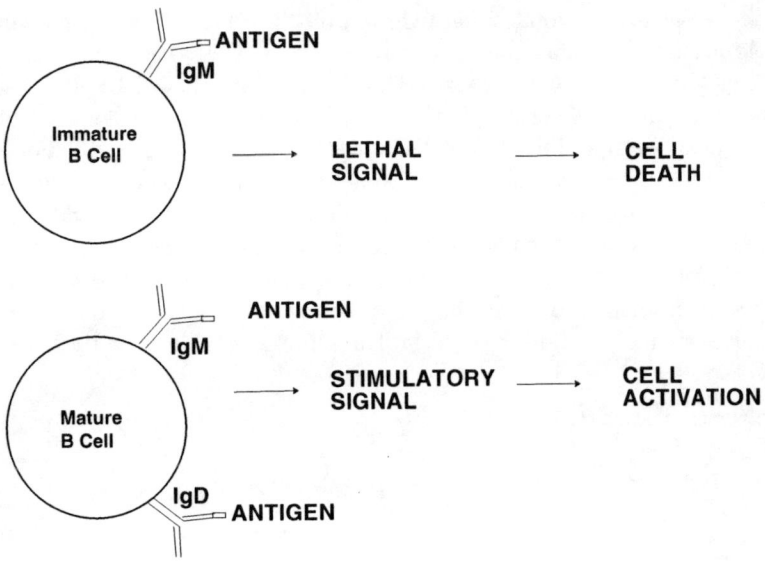

Figure 16-1
Mechanism for B cell clonal deletion.

IMMUNOGEN VS. TOLEROGEN

If an antigen induces activation of a B cell, it is called an *immunogen*. If an antigen does not activate a B cell, it is called a *tolerogen*. Tolerogens induce B cell clonal anergy.

A B cell recognizes an antigen via the antigen-specific immunoglobulin molecule. Both immunogens and tolerogens bind to the immunoglobulin receptor. Immunogens and tolerogens are endocytosed and processed to specific antigenic peptides. These peptides are then presented on the B cell surface in association with its MHC class II molecules. Immunogens in association with class II molecules will be specifically recognized by a specific T cell receptor to initiate an interaction between the T cell and B cell. As discussed in Chap. 7, this initial interaction involves the participation of a number of adhesion molecules (LFA-1/ICAM-1) and co-stimulatory molecules (B7-2/CD28 and CD40/CD40L). The function of the co-stimulatory molecules is to activate the B cell to grow and differentiate.

Tolerogens are peptides that induce a block in the activation, growth, and development of B cells into antibody-secreting cells. Therefore, tolerogens induce a state of B cell clonal anergy. Development of a state of B cell anergy can occur for a number of reasons, but it primarily involves a lack of co-stimulatory signals being delivered to the B cell during T cell-B cell interaction. For example, as shown in Fig. 16-2, if a B cell either does not express enough B7-2 or CD40 on its surface or cannot find a Th cell to interact with to provide co-stimulation, it does not become activated, even though antigen bound to its immunoglobulin receptor and was endocytosed and processed to a peptide fragment for presentation to a Th cell. Expression of co-stimulatory signals on the B cell becomes the rate-limiting step in determining whether or not a B cell will

B CELL ACTIVATION

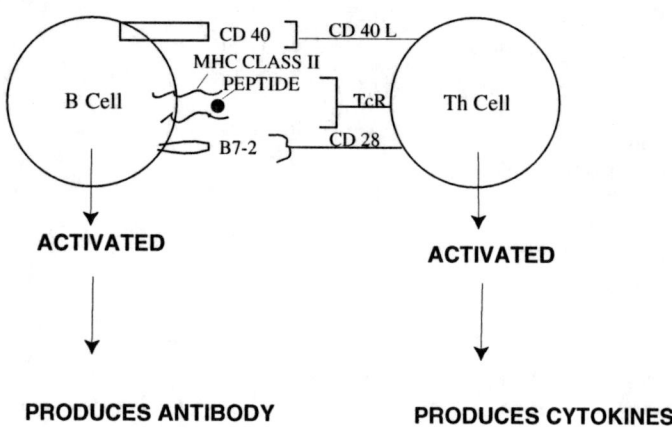

B CELL ANERGY

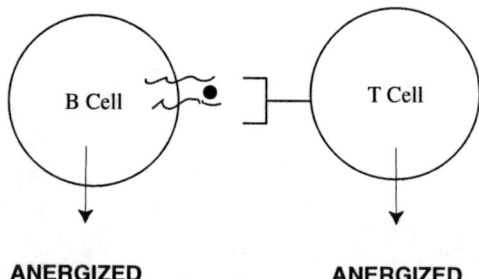

Figure 16-2
Lack of co-stimulatory signals produces a tolerogenic response in a B cell.

become activated to receive signals from the cytokines released by activated Th cells. If the B cell does not receive the co-stimulatory signals, it becomes quiescent and, thus, anergic.

B CELL-ASSOCIATED AUTOIMMUNE DISEASES

These diseases are caused by either the deposition of soluble immune complexes composed of antibody and antigen on blood vessel walls in the body or damage to critical organ tissues by the binding of antibody to tissue-associated molecules and followed by complement-mediated cell lysis.

If the B cell does become activated after binding molecules normally present in the body, it will secrete antibodies against these "self" molecules, with subsequent development of a B cell-associated autoimmune disease.

MECHANISMS FOR BREAKING B CELL TOLERANCE

Molecular mimicry
Polyclonal B cell activation
Polyclonal T cell activation
Exposure of "hidden" self antigens

MOLECULAR MIMICRY

This occurs when antibodies produced against a foreign antigen cross-react with "self" antigens.

Some "self" antigens may cross-react with immunoglobulin produced by a B cell that belongs to a clone of B cells that initially responded to a foreign antigen. These B cells react against the foreign antigen, produce antibodies that are able to capture foreign antigen, and also cross-react with self antigens (Fig. 16-3). This form of tolerance breaking is called *molecular mimicry*. For example, antibodies that are made against streptococcus may cross-react with molecules expressed on the surface of cells of the heart. The resulting heart cell damage that occurs produces the clinical condition known as *rheumatic fever*.

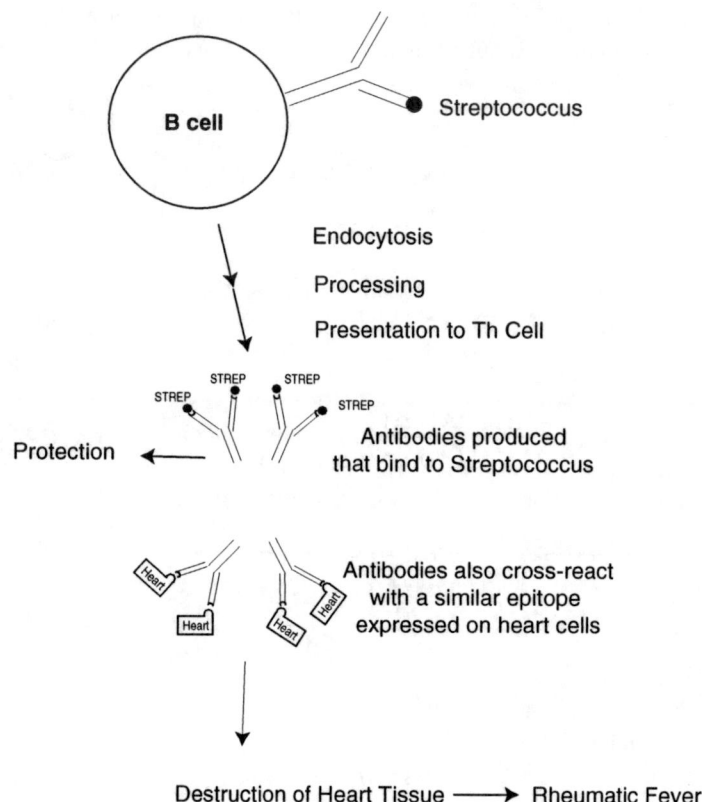

Figure 16-3
Molecular mimicry.

POLYCLONAL B CELL ACTIVATION

This process activates an anergic B cell via a mechanism that does not involve the specific activation of the B cell by the binding of antigen to the immunoglobulin receptor but involves the nonspecific activation of the B cell by nonspecific multivalent antigens containing multiple repeating structural units, such as bacterial cell wall products (lipopolysaccharide).

Polyclonal B cell activation does not require Th cell cytokines and is, thus, T cell-independent. Therefore, an infection with a bacteria whose cell wall can act as a polyclonal stimulant will induce an anergic B cell to clonally expand because the cell no longer requires co-stimulation in order to become an antibody-producing cell. The polyclonally activated cell will produce antibodies against the self antigen that anergized it originally. Now that antibodies are being produced against the "self" antigen, the antibody will bind to the self antigen and cause damage (Fig. 16-4). Because many different anergic B cells will be activated due to the lack of antigen specificity associated with polyclonal activation, autoantibodies will be produced against the cells of many different organ systems, producing a systemic autoimmune disease as opposed to an organ-specific autoimmune disease. For example, systemic lupus erythematosus may be initially caused by a bacterial infection with the subsequent activation of many different

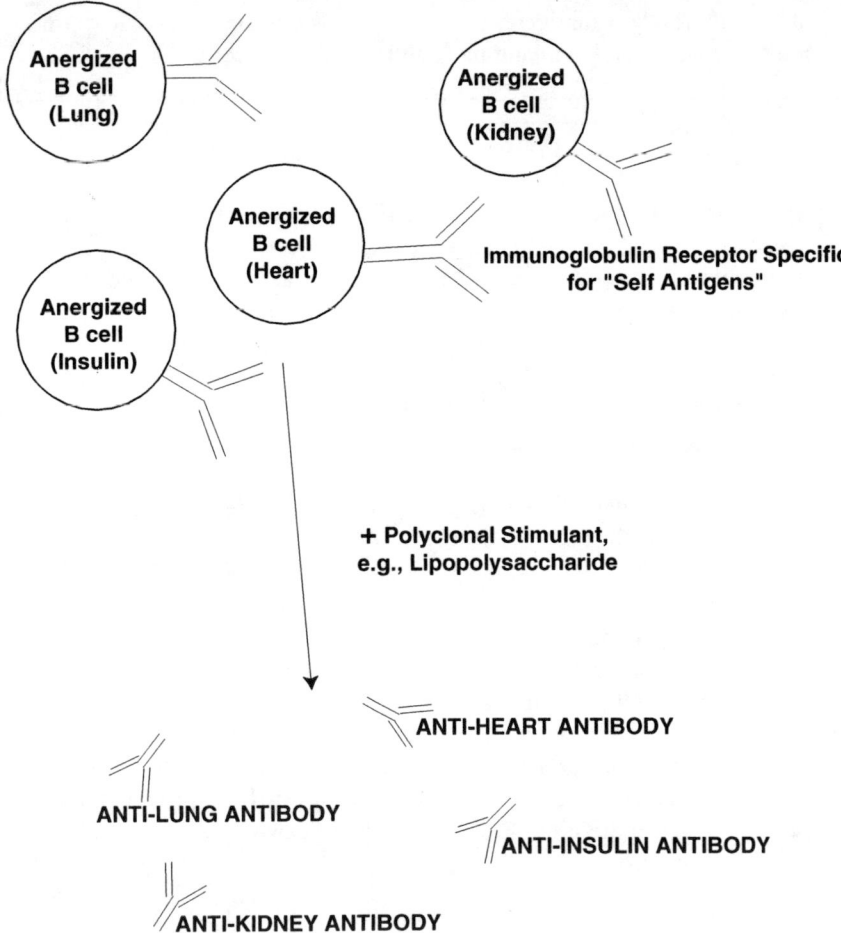

Figure 16-4
Polyclonal B cell activation breaks B cell tolerance.

anergic B cells that become activated to produce antibodies that recognize many different self antigens.

Polyclonal B cell activation may also induce the expression of co-stimulatory molecules on anergic B cells to enable them to successfully interact with Th cells. In this manner, upregulated B7-2 and/or CD40 will make these cells more likely to activate interacting Th cells and also receive Th cell contact-mediated and cytokine-mediated help.

POLYCLONAL T CELL ACTIVATION

This is a process whereby T cells become activated by a polyclonal activator, such as a superantigen. Activated T cells clonally expand and provide cell contact- and cytokine-mediated signals to B cells.

SUPERANTIGENS

Superantigens are molecules derived from bacteria and other pathogens that bind to class II MHC on antigen-presenting cells at sites that are different from the "groove" sites where processed antigenic peptides bind. Thus, superantigens are presented to T cells in an MHC-unrestricted manner and are only presented to T cells expressing a T cell receptor possessing a specific variable β gene product. Thus, many T cells are activated in an antigen-nonspecific and MHC-unrestricted manner.

B cell anergy is partially due to the selection of Th cells in the thymus that do not react against self proteins. However, some T cells escape thymic selection and become anergized in the periphery as was discussed in Chap. 5. These T cells cannot be activated in an antigen-specific manner but can be activated nonspecifically by superantigens. The activated Th cells will express an increased level of CD40L, a molecule that is critical for providing a co-stimulatory activation signal to the B cell through its interaction with CD40 on the B cell. Activated Th cells will also produce cytokines. In this manner, many different anergic B cells can be nonspecifically activated by the interaction of CD40 on the B cell with CD40L on an activated Th cell. The secreted cytokines provide the necessary second signal to drive the B cells to clonally expand and differentiate into antibody-secreting cells.

EXPOSURE OF "HIDDEN" SELF ANTIGENS

This is a process whereby self antigens that are not normally exposed on the exterior of cells are exposed and act as "foreign" antigens, since they have never been seen by immune cells (either B or T) and, therefore, act as immunogens.

Self antigens that do not normally expose themselves to the outside of the cell may actually act as "foreign" antigens if they are ever exposed to the cell's exterior. Remember that some B cells and Th cells have never encountered these molecules before and, therefore, have not been deleted in the thymus, deleted in peripheral germinal centers, or anergized. For example, myelin basic proteins are a major component of Schwann cells and oligodendrocytes but are not normally expressed on the cell surface. In a nerve injury, however, myelin basic proteins are exposed to the cell's exterior and are then recognized as "non-self" because they have never been seen by the immune system before. Thus, *non-self* is a misleading term, since myelin basic proteins are indeed a part of "self." Nonetheless, it is a term that is often used to describe immunogens vs. nonimmunogens. Thus, both B cells and Th cells can be activated upon exposure to myelin basic proteins, and B cells can differentiate into antibody-producing cells. The antibody produced can then bind to myelin basic proteins exposed on injured nerve cells, which activates a number of mechanisms for cell destruction. As a consequence, the nerve may either never repair or be denuded of its protective covering that allows for the fast conductance of nerve impulses. If the latter happens, multiple sclerosis can develop.

TRANSPLANTATION

·

- **Transplant Rejection**
- **Tissue Compatibility**
- **Laws of Transplantation**
- **Histocompatibility Antigens**
- **Graft vs. Host Disease**
- **Mediators of Rejection**
- **Influences on Transplant Success**
- **Immunosuppression**

· · · · · · · · · · · ·

TRANSPLANT REJECTION

Transplant rejection is graft failure resulting from recipient antibodies and cells directed against donor cells.

Transplantation, for the purpose of replacing a diseased organ with a healthy donor organ, represents an increasingly active field in modern medical practice, as our understanding of the immunological aspects of transplantation continues to grow. Transplantation, together with autoimmunity and hypersensitivity reactions discussed earlier (Chaps. 12, 13, and 16), represent situations that involve or have the potential to involve, in the case of transplantation, adverse side effects of an immune system that has evolved to recognize and protect us from harmful pathogens. With regard to transplantation, those adverse side effects sometimes result in graft failure due to an immunologically mediated event termed *rejection*.

TISSUE COMPATIBILITY

The concept of tissue compatibility (i.e., the need for donor and recipient tissues to be "compatible" in order for a transplant to be accepted) was appreciated as early as the beginning of the 20th century. In a series of studies involving the transplantation of tumors and later skin grafts between mice, it became apparent that successful tissue transplantation depended upon genetic similarity of donor and recipient (Table 17-1).

Tissues transplanted between genetically identical animals, also known as *syngeneic* transplants or *isografts*, are virtually always accepted. In contrast, transplants performed between two subjects belonging to the same species who are genetically nonidentical, termed *allogeneic* transplants or *allografts*, invariably undergo rejection. Transplants performed between donor and recipient who belong to different species are known as *xenogeneic* transplants or *xenografts* and are promptly rejected.

Allogeneic transplants or allografts bear allogeneic or foreign major and minor histocompatibility antigens; whereas *syngeneic transplants* or isografts bear genetically identical or "self" major and minor histocompatibility antigens.

LAWS OF TRANSPLANTATION

The laws of transplantation are as follows.

Transplants are accepted between members of a highly inbred genetic strain (haplotype) or animals that are genetically identical (i.e., identical twins).

Transplants are rejected between members of different haplotype or animals that are genetically *non*identical.

Transplants are accepted from parental haplotype A or B to an F_1 (A×B) progeny, but transplants in the reverse direction are rejected.

TABLE 17-1
TYPES OF TRANSPLANTS

TRANSPLANT	GRAFT	DONOR/RECIPIENT
Syngeneic	Isograft	Genetically identical (i.e., identical twins)
Allogeneic	Allograft	Genetically nonidentical members of the same species
Xenogeneic	Xenograft	Belong to different species

HISTOCOMPATIBILITY ANTIGENS

Regarding the issue of genetic similarity between transplant donor and recipient (i.e., *histocompatibility*), early observations on transplant outcome led to the identification of a set of genes whose co-dominant expression elicits vigorous rejection responses in the case of allogeneic transplants. That set of genes has come to be characterized as the *major histocompatibility complex* or *MHC*, the subject of Chap. 6.

It is important to realize that many target antigens exist in cases of graft rejection. The MHC represents the most critical set of genes encoding such cell surface antigens; however, several genetic loci or areas of the MHC have yet to be mapped and defined. Furthermore, another set of genes, encoding *the minor histocompatibility antigens*, may play a very important role in transplant outcome as well. These genes have been less well characterized compared with those encoded by the MHC and generally are believed to play a weaker role in graft rejection events.

In order for a graft to be accepted, the recipient must share an identical complement of donor genes. For example, donor strain A or B into a strain A×B recipient would result in graft acceptance, since both strain A and B genes would be shared by the A×B recipient (Fig. 17-1). In the case of donor tissue from strain A×B transplanted into either strain A or B recipient, the outcome would be graft rejection, since recipient A has donor A genes but not B genes and recipient B has donor B but not A genes.

GRAFT VS. HOST DISEASE

This disease occurs when an immunologically competent foreign graft containing T cells reacts against the MHC antigens of an immunologically compromised host.

In general, concerns regarding the outcome of transplantation represent a one-way street, namely the potential of the immune system of a transplant recipient or host to reject a transplant. An interesting reversal of the direction of the immune response occurs, however, when *immunocompetent cells* (i.e., spleen cells) are transplanted into a host whose immune system is not functioning properly (i.e., irradiated) and is, therefore, immunosuppressed (Fig. 17-2). In this case, a phenomenon known as *graft vs. host disease* ensues, where the immunocompetent graft directs an immunological assault against the host, sometimes with fatal consequences. Graft vs. host disease is, therefore, of particular concern in

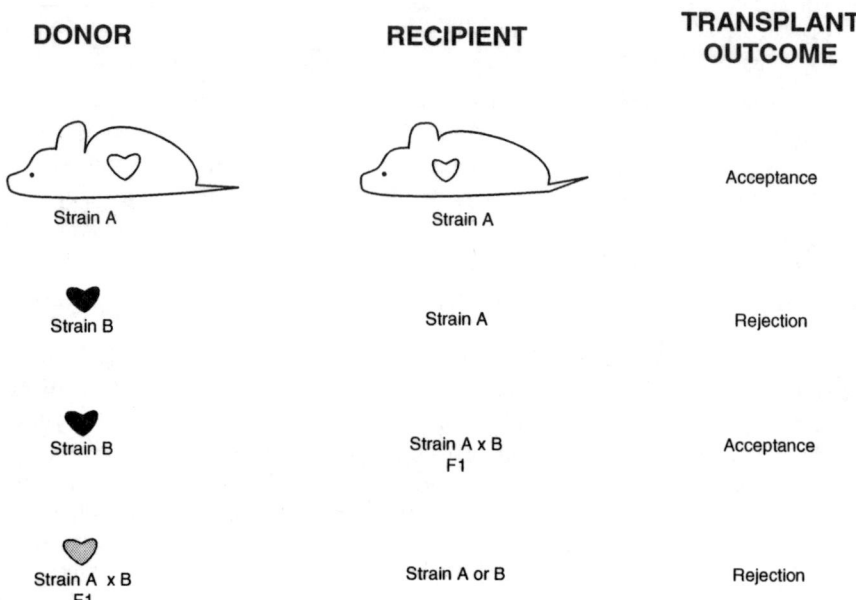

Figure 17-1
Transplant outcome.

cases of bone marrow transplantation, where immunocompetent T cells in the graft tissue can direct a graft rejection response against the cell surface MHC antigens of a frequently immunocompromised recipient or host.

MEDIATORS OF REJECTION

Several components of the immune system are known to mediate graft rejection (Table 17-2).

First, we will consider antibody-mediated graft cell destruction (Fig. 17-3, A), where antibodies specific for graft cell MHC antigens may be elicited with $CD4^+$ T cell help generated in response to foreign graft MHC class II molecules. In the presence of complement, these antigraft antibodies would be capable of lysing (i.e., killing) graft target cells. In the case of cell-mediated graft destruction, at least two scenarios may be considered (Fig. 17-3, B and C). In the first, foreign graft MHC class II molecules stimulate host T-helper cells to provide "help" to host $CD8^+$ T cytotoxic cells, which then may exert lytic action directly

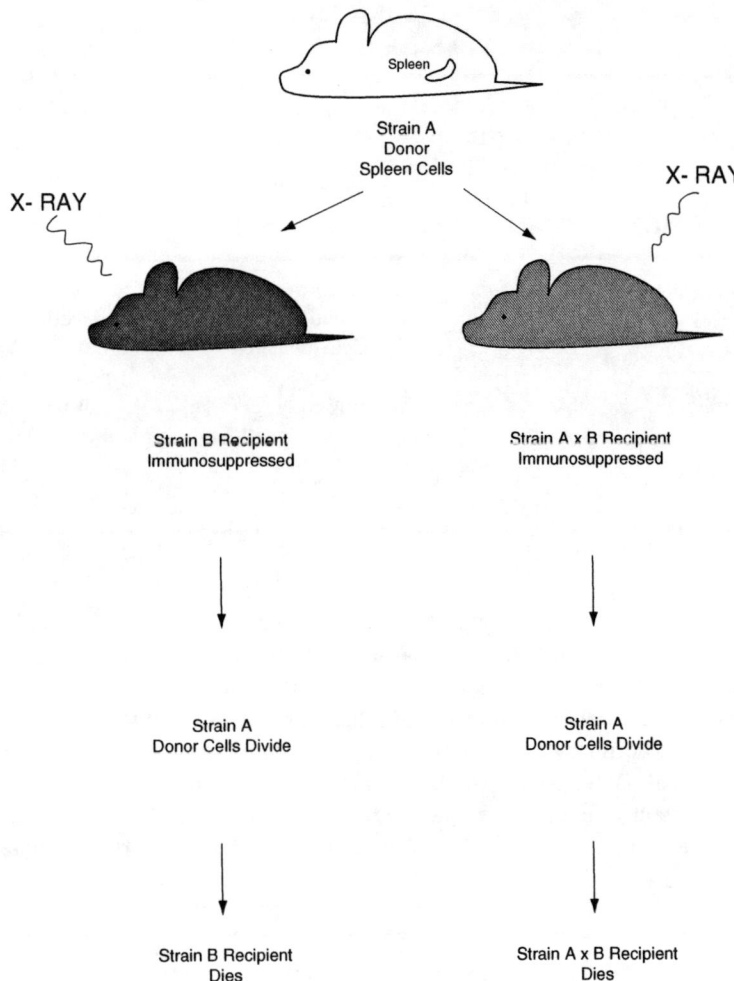

Figure 17-2
Graft vs. host disease.

via recognition of foreign graft MHC class I molecules. Alternatively, stimulated host T helper cells may aid macrophages in an MHC-independent fashion to produce molecules capable of destroying graft cells.

Graft rejection has come to be regarded as being largely cell-mediated, with the T lymphocyte the primary effector cell. This fact is not surprising if one considers Fig. 17-3 again and observes the central role occupied by the T cell. In

TABLE 17-2
TYPES OF REJECTION

REJECTION	ONSET AND DURATION POST-TRANSPLANT	MECHANISM	GRAFT
Hyperacute	Minutes to hours	Preformed antibodies	Xenograft; second set rejection
Acute	Days	Cell-mediated	Allograft with MHC disparity
Chronic	Months	Antibody and/or cell-mediated	Allograft with minor histocompatibility antigen disparity

addition to the cytotoxic T cell, both antibody-mediated and macrophage-mediated graft destruction rely upon T cell help. Antibody-mediated graft destruction, a feature of hyperacute rejection events, also plays an important role in a special situation termed *second set* rejection. In this case, a transplant recipient is retransplanted due to primary graft failure, and upon encounter with the graft's foreign antigens or alloantigens to which the host was previously exposed, the host's immune system generates a hyperacute rejection response. This response consists of preformed cytotoxic antibodies formed during the host's first encounter with graft antigens.

INFLUENCES ON TRANSPLANT SUCCESS

Several factors affect the outcome of tissue transplantation, notably the degree of histocompatibility between donor and recipient.

Fortunately, the availability of reagents specific for cell surface proteins encoded by the MHC has permitted a high degree of cross-matching of donor and recipient where possible prior to transplantation. *Tissue typing/cross-matching* is the identification of the MHC type of transplant donor and recipient to optimize genetic similarity or match prior to transplant. This method (discussed in Chap. 6) and consequently transplant outcome will continue to improve as more MHC loci are characterized and reagents recognizing the products of these gene loci are

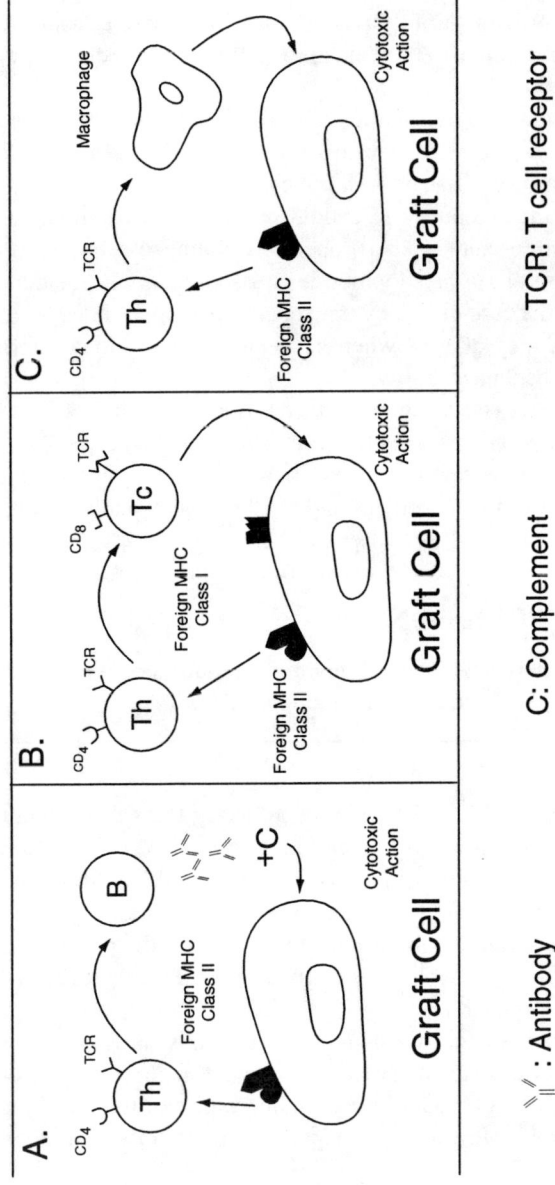

Figure 17-3
Mediators of rejection. (A) Antibody-mediated graft cell destruction. (B) and (C) Cell-mediated graft cell destruction.

prepared. Equally important in cross-matching transplant donor and recipient is the knowledge of *prior sensitization* or foreign antigen encounter by a prospective transplant recipient. Events such as blood transfusion and pregnancy prior to transplant, as well as previous transplants, all may jeopardize transplant success and result in responses similar to hyperacute or second set rejection, a rapid and vigorous reaction.

Of critical importance to transplant success and viability is the degree of *tissue* or *organ preservation* prior to grafting. *Ischemia time*, defined as the time during which the donor organ has been deprived of its proper blood supply, drastically affects transplant outcome and should be kept to a minimum. Ischemia time is particularly important for the proper functioning of kidney, heart, and liver transplants, where organ preservation is an issue. Indeed, considerations of organ preservation in the case of kidney transplants are compounded by the availability of cadaveric kidney donors, where ischemia time and longer-term organ preservation affect transplant viability.

Interestingly, there exist a few sites in the body (central nervous system, reproductive tract) that are considered relatively "*immune privileged*" in terms of their vulnerability to an immune response. These sites generally lack lymphatic drainage and express few MHC antigens and are therefore weakly immunogenic.

IMMUNOSUPPRESSION

Immunosuppression is a generally impaired immune response, with increased susceptibility to infection and malignancies.

The consideration of the various factors affecting transplant outcome now turns to a discussion of a subject of tremendous importance not only to recipient selection but also to long-term transplant recipient care and management, namely the issue of often associated *immunosuppression*. Since graft rejection is provoked by an undesirable but healthy immune response on the part of the host, it is imperative for favorable transplant outcome that the transplant recipient be in some way immunosuppressed.

Immunosuppression of the transplant recipient falls into one of two categories, either suppression targeted specifically toward donor antigen or targeted nonspecifically, resulting in broader immunocompromise of the transplant recipient. Means of achieving both antigen-nonspecific and -specific immunosuppression are listed in Table 17-3.

Total *lymphoid irradiation*, while infrequently used today, effectively eliminates the host immune response, resulting in graft survival, albeit profound im-

TABLE 17-3
TYPES OF IMMUNOSUPPRESSION

ANTIGEN-NONSPECIFIC	ANTIGEN-SPECIFIC
Lymphoid irradiation	Anti-graft antibodies
Antilymphocyte globulins	Anti-TCR antibodies
Antimetabolite drugs–azathioprine	Tolerance
Steroids–prednisone	Central: *in utero*/neonatal by clonal deletion
Immunosuppressive agents– cyclosporine A	Peripheral: in adult by Anergy Suppression Deletion

munosuppression. More frequent approaches to cripple the transplant recipient's immune system have included the use of *anti-lymphocyte globulins*, such as OKT-3, directed against the CD3 component of the human T cell receptor, which serves to inhibit T cell-mediated responses. *Antimetabolite* drugs, such as azathioprine, inhibit nucleotide synthesis and result in suppressing the proliferative capacity of rapidly dividing cells, such as lymphocytes recently recruited to participate in an immune response. Such drugs are frequently used in combination with *steroids*, such as prednisone, which is broadly immunosuppressive by inhibiting lymphocyte function, as well as a drug called *cyclosporine A*, which more specifically inhibits T cell expression of cytokine effector molecules. A triple regimen consisting of azathioprine, prednisone, and cyclosporine A is commonly used post-transplant to manage heart and kidney transplant recipients.

Such effective immunosuppressive measures, due to their broad impact on the host's immune system, as well as frequent adverse side effects, have raised the issue of identifying means of suppressing the transplant rejection response in a more antigen-specific way. It is hoped that such antigen-specific means of immunosuppression, though still in their infancy, will impact less on the host's immune system and result in fewer side effects associated with multiple drug use. One strategy considered in antigen-specific immunosuppression is to employ antibodies directed against graft antigens, such as MHC alloantigens, which results in a prolongation of graft survival known as *enhancement*. The mechanism by which *anti-graft antibodies* promote transplant survival is currently under investigation. Another donor antigen-specific approach to immunsuppression, still in an experimental phase of study, is the use of *anti-T cell receptor* (*TCR*) *antibodies* to block host T cells specific for allogeneic MHC. This kind of therapy implies a detailed knowledge not only of which MHC alloantigens are expressed on each graft, but also which antigen epitopes are critical for generating host T cell help during the alloimmune response.

Antibody therapy, whether donor antigen-specific or -nonspecific, due to its passive nature, usually requires chronic administration. Associated with long-term antibody therapy is the adverse sensitization of the individual receiving these antibodies, which are usually raised in nonhuman species. These antibodies, therefore, act as alloantigens due to foreign isotope sequences and as such have the potential to provoke anti-antibody responses in the recipient. Clearly, such a situation renders antibody therapy of limited long-term value.

In the face of these therapeutic difficulties, an appealing strategy aimed at inducing donor antigen-specific immunosuppression is the concept of *tolerance*, defined here as specific, acquired, long-lasting immunological unresponsiveness. Tolerance to "self" antigens occurs very early in life, during fetal and neonatal development, as discussed in Chap. 16. Self-tolerance or *central tolerance* is principally acquired by negative selection or elimination of potentially self-reactive T cell clones during thymic development. Negative selection in the thymus is characterized by programmed cell death in a process referred to as *clonal deletion*.

Tolerance to prospective donor alloantigens, however, raises the issue of how to achieve tolerance in the adult transplant recipient long after central or self-tolerance has been achieved. Issues surrounding how to establish *peripheral* (nonthymic) tolerance form the basis of many experimental studies in the fields of transplantation and autoimmunity today. While still at their inception, these studies aim to elucidate how prior oral or intravenous administration of donor allo-MHC antigens, in the case of transplantation, sometimes achieves a tolerant state in the transplant recipient. Also under investigation are the doses of antigen required to induce tolerance, described as either *low zone* or *high zone*, depending upon the relative doses of antigen needed to achieve it. Route of administration and antigen dose aside, experimental observations published to date have indicated that *tolerance* to donor allo-MHC antigens may be established by a combination of active *suppression* of the recipient immune response and/or failure to respond to foreign antigen mediated by either T cell *clonal deletion* or *anergy*. Anergy may be defined as the absence of an immune response due to loss of cell function or "immune paralysis" and may be reversible. Future transplant therapy awaits clarification of these issues.

NEUROENDOCRINIMMUNOLOGY

•

- Endocrine-Immune Autoregulatory Loop
- Immune Cell Expression of Receptors for Neuroendocrine Hormones
- Neuro-Immune Autoregulatory Loop
- Immune Cell Expression of Receptors for Norepinephrine
- Modulation of Immune Cell Function by Opioid Neuropeptides
- Immune Cell Production and Secretion of Neuroendocrine Molecules
- Immune Cell Communication with the Central Nervous System (CNS)
- Microglia
- Cytokine Production by Cells Residing in the CNS

•   •   •   •   •   •   •   •   •   •   •   •

In recent years, a number of scientific studies have indicated that mechanisms exist for the nervous, endocrine, and immune systems to communicate with each other. These studies show that cells from all three systems appear to share a number of the same receptors for neurotransmitters, hormones, and cytokines in addition to synthesizing and secreting some of the same molecules, such as cytokines and neuropeptides. Therefore, it appears that each system can modulate cellular functions associated with either itself or with the other two systems. What appears to trigger this communication among the systems is the appearance of antigen in the body. Fig. 18-1 shows the neuroendocrine-immune pathways that are triggered by antigen. These pathways will be described in detail in the following sections.

Shortly after the appearance of antigen in the body, an immune response begins, resulting in the synthesis and release of cytokines from activated immune cells into the circulation. As circulating cytokine levels increase, a change occurs in the firing rate of neurons within the hypothalamus to trigger two different pathways from the brain to peripheral lymphoid organs. One pathway involves the

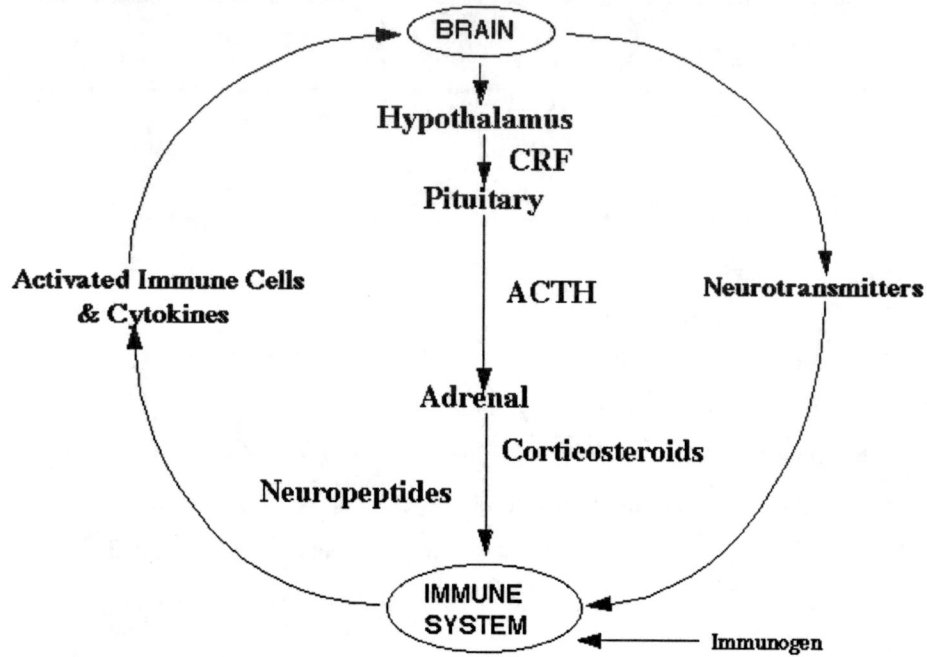

Figure 18-1
Cytokines are produced by cells that reside within the CNS to either protect or damage neurons/glia.

release of corticotropin-releasing factor (CRF) from the hypothalamus, while the other pathway involves the activation of the sympathetic nervous system (SNS).

ENDOCRINE-IMMUNE AUTOREGULATORY LOOP

Antigen → immune cell activation → IL-1 release → hypothalamus → CRF release → pituitary → ACTH release → adrenal cortex → corticosteroid release → immunosuppression → decreased IL-1 release → decreased corticosteroid release

---

In the first pathway, the release of interleukin (IL)-1 from the immune system triggers the hypothalamus to release CRF to stimulate the expression of pro-opiomelanocortin (POMC) in the pituitary gland. The expressed POMC is enzymatically converted within the pituitary into either the endocrine hormone adrenocorticotropin (ACTH) or the neuropeptide β-endorphin. The newly synthesized ACTH is released from the pituitary to induce the secretion of corticosteroids from the adrenal cortex to act directly on immune cells to suppress their activity. Interestingly, all of the intermediate molecules involved in corticosteroid release, namely CRF, β-endorphin and ACTH, are also able to act directly on immune cells to modulate their level of activity. The action of these intermediate molecules on immune cell function can be either enhancing or suppressive, depending on their concentration and the immune cell type affected.

Eventually, the activated immune system returns to a baseline level of activity because the pathway described above begins to generate an autoregulatory loop. First, the corticosteroids suppress the release of IL-1 from activated immune cells. The release of IL-1 is also diminished by the eventual removal of antigen by phagocytic cells, resulting in the loss of the antigen trigger for immune cell activation. In this manner, both of these mechanisms remove the IL-1 signal to the hypothalamus. However, the body does not want the immune system to get too suppressed (remember, some effector immune cells still need to produce antibody or kill infected cells). For this reason, the corticosteroids also feed back to both the hypothalamus and pituitary to inhibit CRF release and ACTH secretion, respectively. The resulting decrease in CRF and ACTH ultimately results in a decrease in the release of corticosteroids from the adrenal cortex and, thus, removal of the suppressive signal to immune cells.

IMMUNE CELL EXPRESSION OF RECEPTORS FOR NEUROENDOCRINE HORMONES

Immune cells express receptors for CRF, ACTH, and glucocorticoids. Therefore, immune cell activity can be modulated by any of the molecules released along the endocrine-immune autoregulatory loop.

It is interesting to note that the release of many of the endocrine hormones described above can be stimulated by stress situations. If stress occurs before an immune response, antigen may not be able to activate immune cells that have been suppressed by corticosteroids. On the other hand, if stress occurs during an immune response, the level of corticosteroids may be higher and remain elevated for a longer period of time, resulting in prolonged immune suppression of effector cell functions.

NEURO-IMMUNE AUTOREGULATORY LOOP

Antigen → immune cell activation → IL-1 release → hypothalamus → CRF release → activation of the SNS → release of NE → immunosuppression/immunoenhancement → decreased IL-1 release → decreased SNS activity

The second pathway for communication from the brain to the periphery involves the activation of the sympathetic nervous system (SNS). The sympathetic nervous system, as part of the autonomic nervous system, maintains a constant internal environment for the body by regulating the activities of a number of organ systems that are not under voluntary, conscious control. The major neurotransmitter released by the sympathetic nervous system is norepinephrine (NE). As in the immune-endocrine pathway, the release of IL-1 from the immune system triggers the hypothalamus to release CRF. However, as opposed to stimulating ACTH release from the pituitary, CRF stimulates activation of the SNS and release of NE. Also, cytokines released from immune cells may cross into the central nervous system and stimulate other pathways that lead to activation of the SNS. Sympathetic nerve fibers containing NE are found in primary and secondary lymphoid organs. In the spleen and lymph nodes these fibers end at a point adjacent to CD4+ T cells and CD8+ T cells located within the periarteriolar lymphoid sheath (PALS) and to macrophages located within the marginal zone. In contrast, sympathetic nerve fibers rarely end on B cells.

IMMUNE CELL EXPRESSION OF RECEPTORS FOR NOREPINEPHRINE

Binding studies on resting immune cells show the presence of high affinity β-adrenergic receptors that are of the β-2-subtype, exclusively, that can bind norepinephrine.

Norepinephrine sends signals to cells by binding to either α- or β-adrenergic receptors. The number of receptors expressed by immune cells seems to be greatest on CD8+ cells, followed by macrophages, B cells, and CD4+ cells. By binding to these receptors on immune cells, NE is able to modulate their ability to function. The modulatory effect induced by NE on immune cells is usually inhibitory, but this inhibition may be dependent on the way cells are activated (soluble vs. particulate antigens), the cytokines produced by activated cells (IL-2 vs. IL-4), and/or the specific immune response being modulated (antibody production vs. cell proliferation). For example, stimulation of the β-2-adrenergic receptor expressed on Th1 cells appears to inhibit the production of IL-2 and interferon-γ, but it does not appear to affect IL-4 production by Th2 cells. Another example is that β-2-adrenergic receptor stimulation of B cells appears to render more antigen-specific B cells capable of going on to make specific antibody against both soluble and particulate antigens.

Eventually, however, the activated immune system returns to a baseline level of activity because of a mechanism similar to the autoregulatory loop described above for the immune-endocrine autoregulatory loop. Basically, anti-gen removal decreases the production of IL-1, which decreases CRF release and, consequently, SNS activation.

Activation of either of the two pathways, involving either corticosteroid or NE release, probably occurs at different times during the course of an immune response. For example, norepinephrine seems to affect immune responses early in the response because nerve fibers are in the direct vicinity of responding cells, thus allowing for initial signals to be delivered quickly, efficiently, and effec-tively. In contrast, an increase in corticosteroid levels occurs later in the response, at a time when the response needs to be dampened.

The role of the neuroendocrine-immune autoregulatory loop in the etiology or progression of disease states is circumstantial at present. For example, an age-related decline in the number of sympathetic nerve fibers going to lymphoid organs may increase the level of susceptibility of an older person to viral and bacterial infections, while, on the other hand, an age-related decline in immune cell function may induce behavioral and cognitive dysfunctions associated with aging. Although these possibilities are speculative, they emphasize the need for a better understanding of the mechanisms by which one system influences the func-tioning of the other to either maintain homeostasis or influence the etiology or progression of nervous and immune disease states.

MODULATION OF IMMUNE CELL FUNCTION BY OPIOID NEUROPEPTIDES

Concomitant with ACTH and norepinephrine release is the release of endorphin and enkephalin opioid neuropeptides, respectively. Immune cells express high affinity receptors for the opioid neuropeptides.

Endorphins are released as a consequence of POMC metabolism, and enkephalins co-reside with norepinephrine in sympathetic nerve terminals as a precursor molecule named preproenkephalin. In addition to being secreted by sympathetic nerve endings, enkephalins are also released by the adrenal medulla. Endorphins and enkephalins are neuropeptides that belong to a family of opioid peptides, consisting also of dynorphins. Immunocompetent cells express recep-tors for these neuropeptides that transduce signals to either enhance or suppress immune functions, depending on the subtype and concentration of neuropeptide involved in the response (Met-enkephalin vs. Leu-enkephalin) and the cell type affected. For example, ultralow concentrations of Met-enkephalin appear to sup-press the ability of B cells to make antibody, while high concentrations of Met-enkephalin may enhance the ability of T cells to make cytokines.

IMMUNE CELL PRODUCTION AND SECRETION OF NEUROENDOCRINE MOLECULES

Although endorphins, enkephalins, CRF, and ACTH have been classically thought to be released only by cells of the neuroendocrine system to influence predominantly neuroendocrine cell function, more recent studies have shown that activated immune cells themselves can synthesize these neuropeptides and hormones.

Two major immune cell sources for these peptides and hormones are the CD4+ T cell and macrophage. Thus, neuropeptide and hormone release by either the nervous system or immune system can modulate the cellular functions of both systems.

IMMUNE CELL COMMUNICATION WITH THE CENTRAL NERVOUS SYSTEM (CNS)

Until recently, the CNS has been considered an immune-privileged site. This meant that the CNS was thought to be devoid of immune cells. However, recent studies show that activated immune cells in the periphery can traverse the blood-brain barrier (BBB) and reside in the CNS to influence the development and progression of certain CNS-related diseases.

Either the release of cytokines by activated immune cells or the movement of activated cells themselves into the CNS provides a mechanism by which the immune system can communicate with the CNS to signal that immune homeostasis has been threatened. This communication may result in the immune system either enlisting "help" from the nervous system to up- or down-modulate peripheral immune cell activity, triggering the development of autoimmune disorders in the CNS, or inducing neural events associated with sickness behavior precipitated by bacterial and viral infections.

The mechanism by which immune cells from the periphery enter the CNS to cause autoimmune disorders such as multiple sclerosis is only beginning to be understood. Essentially, as depicted in Fig. 18-2, cytokines released by activated immune cells appear to increase the permeability of the BBB to allow for the passage of peripheral immune cells into the brain that release cytokines to induce within the CNS potentiation of the immune response and/or neuronal damage. For example, CD4+ Th1 cells in the periphery that are specific for the recogni-

Autoimmune-Mediated Damage in the CNS

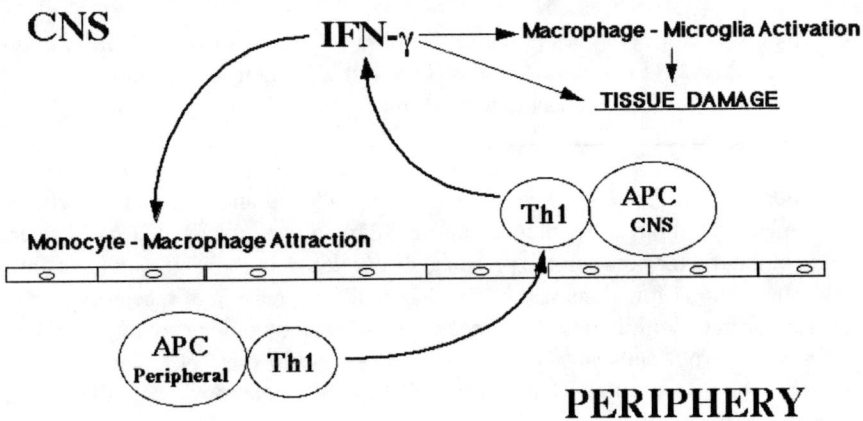

Figure 18-2
Th1 cells activated in the periphery can cross the blood-brain barrier to cause damage in the CNS.

tion of myelin basic protein (MBP) can be detected within the CNS at a time that correlates with the induction of the demyelinating disease multiple sclerosis. These CD4+ Th1 cells initially respond to nerve damage in the periphery where the once hidden MBP acts as an antigen. MBP-specific CD4+ Th1 cells become activated in the periphery to release cytokines that increase the permeability of the BBB, allowing for the Th1 cells to traverse the BBB and become reactivated in the CNS by myelin basic proteins presented to them by *microglia*.

MICROGLIA

Microglia are bone marrow-derived antigen-presenting cells that reside in the CNS.

Upon activation, these Th1 cells release interferon-γ and tumor necrosis factor α to activate more microglia to present antigen and induce severe nerve damage, respectively. The resulting nerve damage in the CNS along with the demyelination in the periphery eventually result in the characteristic nerve dysfunctions associated with multiple sclerosis.

CYTOKINE PRODUCTION BY CELLS RESIDING IN THE CNS

The presence of cytokines in the CNS reflects not only their production in the periphery and circulation to the CNS, but also their local synthesis by cells residing within the CNS, such as microglia and astrocytes.

As shown in Fig. 18-3, cytokines can be produced and secreted by cells of the immune system to either induce neuronal damage or enhance neuronal repair. The deciding factor between the presence of cytokines in the CNS and their ability to alter cellular functions within the CNS is the expression of receptors for the cytokine on cells within the CNS. Receptors for most cytokines are expressed by a number of CNS cells in a variety of regions within the CNS. For example, receptors for IL-1 are localized to primarily the hippocampus, cerebellum, and hypothalamus, IL-2 receptors are localized to primarily the hippocampus and cerebellum, and IL-6 receptors are associated primarily with astrocytes and the hypothalamus.

Cytokines within the CNS not only affect neuronal damage and repair, but some, such as IL-1, act as endogenous pyrogens, inducing the fever that accompanies inflammatory immune responses. IL-1 has also been reported to enhance

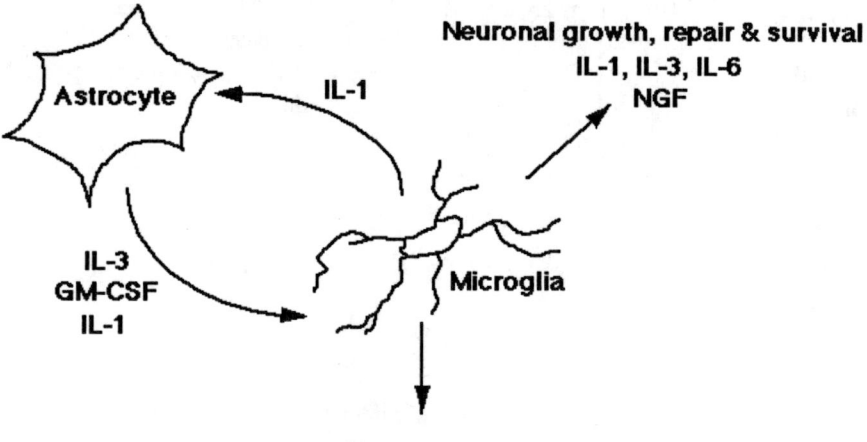

Figure 18-3
Neuro-endocrine-immune connection.

slow wave sleep, enhance opioid receptor binding in the brain, and enhance β-endorphin production in the pituitary. On the other hand, IL-2 alters oligodendrocyte proliferation and inhibits cholinergic activity in various regions of the CNS, while IL-6 acts synergistically with IL-1 in its ability to increase circulating ACTH levels *in vivo*. Thus, cytokines produced outside or within the CNS can potentially influence neuronal, behavioral, and cognitive functions.

The role of the neuroendocrine-immune interrelationship in disease development, dormancy, and progression is currently an area of active research. Since data suggest that immune cell dysfunction plays a role in disease development, dormancy, and progression, it is essential that research be conducted to examine the mechanisms used by the body to either enhance or suppress immune cell function. Conversely, since the cells of the immune system and the cytokines secreted by them play a role in the development and progression of a number of neuroendocrine diseases, it is essential that research be conducted to examine the immune mechanisms used by the body to either enhance or suppress neuroendocrine cell function. By understanding such mechanisms, we will add to our knowledge of neuroendocrine and immune cell function and, more importantly, strengthen our rationales for the development of new approaches to disease prevention and treatment.

· G L O S S A R Y ·

Accessory cell. Cell which aids, but does not directly mediate an adaptive immune response. Includes **antigen presenting cells,** NK, and mast cells.

Acute phase proteins. Serum proteins primarily produced by the liver whose levels increase during acute inflammation or infection. They are an indicator of inflammation and are needed during early phases of acute inflammation.

Adaptive acquired immune response. Clonally selected antigen-specific lymphocytes that respond to an antigen and develop immunological memory.

ADCC (antibody-dependent cell-mediated cytotoxicity). Killing of antibody-coated target cells by effector cells with Fc receptors that recognize the Fc region of the bound antibody. Effectors are NK cells or phagocytic cells which have CD16 or the FcγRIII type of Fc receptor.

Adhesion molecules. Integrins, selectins, members of the immunoglobulin gene superfamily, which mediate binding of lymphoid cells to one another or to the extracellular matrix.

Adjuvant. A substance when mixed with an antigen enhances an immune response.

Affinity maturation. An increase in the affinity of specific antibody for antigen. The antibody is expressed on the cell surface of B cell centrocytes in the basal light zone of germinal centers during a humoral immune response.

Allele. Variant forms of a particular gene at a single locus. Multiple alleles result in **polymorphism**.

Allelic exclusion. Expression of only one allele of a gene. B and T cells express an antigen-binding receptor that recognizes one specific antigen with high affinity.

Allergy. Response to environmental antigen (allergen) due to pre-existing IgE antibody attached to mast cells. An immediate hypersensitivity reaction is produced by mast cell products (histamine, etc.) causing asthma, hay fever, serum sickness, systemic anaphylaxis, or contact dermatitis.

Allogeneic. Two individuals of same species that differ at the MHC (see also **Syngeneic** and **Xenogeneic**).

Allograft. A tissue or cellular transplant between allogeneic individuals. The receipient's T cells will normally react to foreign MHC antigens in the graft unless they are suppressed or are genetically unable.

Allotypes. The different forms of a gene for a particular locus which determines the amino acid composition of the constant regions of Ig H and L chains for each individual.

Alternate pathway. Complement protein C3b binds to the surface of a pathogen and activates C3 convertase → C9. Factors B, D, and properdin are involved to generate the **MAC**. It is a component of innate immunity which can amplify the classical complement pathway.

Anaphylatoxins. C5, C3a, and C4a complement proteins that recruit fluid and inflammatory cells to sites of antigen location. These proteins mediate degranulation of mast cells and basophils.

Anaphylaxis. A systemic allergic reaction caused by the binding of an antigen to IgE on mast cells causing the release of inflammatory mediators (histamine, etc.), which cause circulatory vasodilation, smooth muscle contraction, and suffocation due to tracheal swelling.

Anergy (clonal). Inability of T and B cells to respond to their specific antigen under optimal conditions.

Antibody (immunoglobulin). Plasma proteins produced by plasma cells in response to a specific antigen. Consists of two identical light and heavy chains with specific binding sites on their N-terminal end for a specific site (**epitope**) on the antigen that elicited their production. Surface membrane-bound IgM and IgD antibody is expressed on newly-formed B cells even before they have encountered the specific antigen.

Antigen. Molecule that binds to an antibody or a T cell receptor. **Immunogens** are antigens that induce an antigen-specific immune response.

Antigen-binding site (paratope). Site in the variable (V) domain of an antibody or T cell receptor that binds the **epitope** of an antigen. The complementary determining regions (CDRs 1-3) within the hypervariable loops of both heavy and light chains of antibody molecules are important in determining the structure of the paratope.

Antigen presentation. Whole antigen is degraded into peptide fragments and displayed to a T cell receptor within the groove of a MHC I and/or II molecule.

Antigen presenting cell. Cells which can either process antigen or present already processed antigenic peptides in association with their MHC class II molecules and which possess **co-stimulatory molecules** necessary for lymphocyte activation. Primarily macrophages, dendritic cells, and B cells.

Apoptosis. Cell death resulting from activation of an internal lethal caspase enzyme cascade resulting in nuclear membrane damage, DNA fragmentation, and condensation, culminating in apoptotic body formation. Found in high levels during development of T cells in the thymus and during antibody formation by centrocytes in germinal centers.

Autograft. Tissue graft from one site to another in the same individual.

Autoreactivity. An immune response to self-antigens.

B7 molecules (B7.1:CD80; B7.2:CD86). The main co-stimulatory molecules for CD28 and CTLA-4 on T cells. Related to members of the immunoglobulin gene superfamily.

Basophils. Nonphagocytic granulocyte with Fc_ϵ receptors. Contain large granules with heparin and histamine. Antigen binding to IgE monomer attached to Fc_ϵ receptor triggers degranulation and immediate hypersensitivity response.

B cells. Develop in the bone marrow under the influence of IL-7 and contact-mediated signals delivered by stromal cells. One of three classes of lymphocytes other than T and NK cells. Their antigen-binding receptor is cell surface IgM.

When stimulated, B cells differentiate into plasma cells producing antibody with the same specificity as the original cell surface IgM. As B cells become memory cells, they express IgG antibody on their cell surface.

Bcl-2. An oncogenic protein that prevents apoptosis by inhibiting the conversion of caspase-1 to caspase-3 in the apoptotic pathway. Found on the outer mitochondrial membrane, the endoplasmic reticulum, and nuclear envelope. Also, functions as an ion channel and an adapter or docking protein.

Bone marrow. Site where hematopoietic cells develop in the newborn, as well as white and red blood cells in the adult. B cells develop in the bone marrow and this compartment gives rise to pre-T cells which go to the thymus for selection and maturation.

Bone marrow chimera. Formed by transferring bone marrow from one individual to an irradiated recipient resulting in all hematopoietic elements of donor origin.

Calcineurin. A calmodulin-dependent cytosolic serine/threonine phosphatase that is important in activation of NF-AT (nuclear factor of activated T cells) during T cell activation. Inhibited by the immunosuppressive drugs **cyclosporin A** and FK-506, which form complexes with **immunophilins** (enzymes with peptidyl-prolyl cis-trans isomerase activity) which then binds to and inactivates calcineurin.

Caspases. Part of a series of specific intracellular serine proteases important in the apoptotic pathway. All caspases have cysteine at their active site, require aspartic acid at their cleavage site, and are synthesized as proenzymes.

CD   Clusters of Differentiation (see Appendix 1).

Cell adhesion molecules (CAMs). A class of cell-surface proteins necessary in intercellular adhesion. Include integrins, selectins, and immunoglobulin superfamily.

Cellular immunity. An immune response mediated by antigen specific T cells and other non-specific accessory cells of the immune system. Evolved to protect against intracellular bacteria, viruses, and some cancers, causes graft rejection, and causes graft-versus-host disease.

Centroblasts. Proliferating B blasts found in the dark zone of germinal centers. Somatic hypermutation takes place in them. They give rise to **centrocytes** in the basal light zone.

Centrocytes. Non-proliferating progeny of centroblasts that are located in the light zone of germinal centers. Depending on their interaction with antigen on the surface of follicular dendritic cells, they may mature into plasmablasts, memory B cells, or die via apoptosis.

Chemokine. Low molecular weight polypeptides involved in the directed migration (chemotaxis) and activation of phagocytes and lymphocytes. Very important in inflammation.

Classical complement pathway. Activated by antigen-antibody complexes and involves C1, C4, and C2 in generating C3/C5 convertase.

Clonal selection theory. Adaptive immunity occurs when antigen binds to membrane antibody on B cells or the antigen specific T cell receptor to stimulate these cells to enlarge and divide. These proliferating cells develop into a **clone** of cells with the same specificity as the original responding cells. This clone also gives rise to memory cells. If antigen causes the cells to be killed, it is said to cause **clonal deletion**.

Complementary determining regions (CDRs). Three loops in the terminal end of the variable region of the B cell surface immunoglobulin and T cell receptor that makes contact with the specific ligand. Also called **hypervariable region** because their extreme variability among immunoglobulins and T cell receptors give them their diversity.

Complement system. A group of over 20 serum proteins that act in concert to attack extracellular pathogens. Activated via antigen-antibody binding (**classical** pathway) or spontaneously by C3b binding directly to the surface of a pathogen (**alternate** pathway). Complement coats the pathogen and if C1-9 are bound, it is killed. Also, C3b acts as an **opsonin** facilitating pagocytosis.

Cortex. The outer layer or periphery of an organ.

Co-stimulatory molecules. Molecules on the surface of antigen presenting cells (APC) that may be necessary for lymphocyte activation in addition to antigen binding. T cells require **B7.1 (CD80)** and/or **B7.2 (CD86)** on APCs which bind to **CD28** and **CTLA-4** on the surface of T cells. B cells require **CD40 ligand** on CD4 cells to bind to their **CD40**.

Cyclosporin A (see **Calcineurin**).

Cytokines (see Appendix 2). Proteins produced by cells that have autocrine, paracrine, or endocrine actions on themselves or other cells. Most target cells have specific receptors. **Interleukins (IL)** are cytokines primarily produced by lymphocytes.

D (diversity) gene segment. DNA sequences that join V and J segments in immunoglobulin heavy-chain genes and between the β and δ chain genes in the T cell receptor. They are important in joining these segments during somatic generation of V regions during ontogeny.

Diapedesis. Leukocyte movement between endothelial cells of blood vessels into the tissues. Important in movement of lymphocytes across high endothelial cells lining post-capillary venules in the lymph node deep cortex.

Eosinophils. Leukocytes important in defense against parasites. High levels in immediate hypersensitivity reaction because of their content of histaminase. Activated by IL-5 from Th2 cells.

Epitope (see **Antibody**).

FAS. A member of the TNF family which is expressed on target cells making them targets for killing by FAS-ligand expressing cells.

Follicular dendritic cells. Cells with long dendritic processes which make contact with centrocytes in the germinal center. Contain Fc receptors to hold antigen-antibody complexes for many years.

Germinal centers (2° follicles). In the cortex of lymph nodes, the peripheral white pulp of the spleen, and beneath the epithelial lining in gut-associated lymphoid tissue. They are formed when activated B cells enter **primary follicles**. Consists of a basal dark zone containing both centroblasts and Th cells, and a light zone containing centrocytes, follicular dendritic cells, macrophages, and Th cells. Sites for B cell proliferation, selection, death, and maturation.

Graft-versus-host disease (GVHD). When immunocompetent T cells are injected into an immuno-unresponsive recipient, they react to the recipient's surface MHC antigens and cause a systemic disease (GVHD) affecting the gut, liver, lymphoid tissue, skin, and lungs. Peripheral blood Th cells contained in an allogeneic bone marrow transplant can cause GVHD.

Granulocyte. A leukocyte with cytoplasmic granules such as **neutrophils**, **eosinophils**, and **basophils**. Even though NK cells have granules, they are not usually considered to be granulocytes.

Granzymes A, B. Serine proteases with specificity for aspartic acid. Stored in the granules of cytoxic cells along with perforin. Transferred into target cells through 10-20 nm poly-perforin pores. Activate caspase-3 and thus induces Bcl-2 independent apopotosis.

Gut-associated lymphoid tissue (GALT). Lymphoid tissue associated with the gastrointestinal tract. Includes the palatine, pharyngeal, and lingual tonsils, Peyers patches, appendix, and intraepithelial lymphocytes.

Haplotype. Linked set of **alleles** of genes present on one parental heploid chromosome. One haplotype of MHC genes are inherited from each parent.

Hapten. Low molecular weight molecules that bind antibody, but must be chemically linked to a carrier in order to elicit T cell or antibody responses.

Heavy chain. Each IgG immunoglobulin has 2 identical heavy (H) and light (L) chains. Each H chain has a variable domain (V_H) at the N-terminal end and 3-4 constant (C_H) domains at the C-terminal end. There are 5 major classes (**isotypes**) of heavy chains that each denote a specific function of the antibody molecule.

Helper T cells (Th). A functional class of $CD4^+$ T cells which secrete cytokines necessary in the generation of cell-mediated (Th1) and humoral (Th2) adaptive immune responses. However, not all $CD4^+$ cells are Th cells, as some have been reported to be cytotoxic.

Hematopoiesis. Generation of white and red blood cells, as well as platelets from **hematopoietic stem cells** (HSC). Most HSC reside in the bone marrow and their differentiation requires various growth factors.

High endothelial venules (HEV). Specialized post-capillary venules with a high cuboidal rather than squamous endothelium. Found primarily in the deep cortex of lymph nodes and in the parafollicular area of Peyers patches in the ileum. Circulating lymphocytes migrate through them into the parenchyma of these organs by diapedesis.

Histamine.   An amine stored in mast cell and basophil granules which can cause local blood vessel dilation, increased vascular permeability, and smooth muscle contraction. Released upon antigen (allergen) binding to IgE that is attached to Fc$_\epsilon$ receptors expressed on the surface of these cells.

Histocompatibility.   Individuals whose MHC antigens are identical. Thus, grafts between them will be accepted.

HIV (human immunodeficiency virus).   A retrovirus that infects CD4$^+$ cells and macrophages, causing slow depletion of primarily CD4$^+$ cells to eventually cause acquired immunodeficiency syndrome (AIDS).

HLA (human leukocyte antigen).   The MHC in humans.

Humoral immunity.   Protective immunity mediated by antibody present in the plasma, lymph, and extracellular fluids.

Hypersensitivity.   Systemic exaggerated immune responses upon re-exposure to a particular antigen.

Hypervariable regions (see **Complementary determining regions-CDRs**).

Iccosomes.   Membrane bound immune complexes that fragment off the dendritic processes of follicular dendritic cells. Particularly prominent in a secondary response.

Idiotype.   The distinguishing or antigenic characteristics of the V region of a T cell receptor or antibody molecule. Each idiotype is made up of a series of **idiotopes** (single antigenic determinants).

Immunogen.   A protein recognized by a B cell or T cell antigen receptor which elicits an adaptive immune response.

Immunoglobulin superfamily.   Proteins that contain **immunoglobulin domains** (2 β-pleated sheets joined by an intrachain disulfide bond). Include immunoglobulins, T-cell receptors, MHC molecules, B7 molecules, and some cell adhesion molecules.

Immunophilins   (see **Calcineurin**).

Immunoreceptor tyrosine-based activation motifs (ITAMs).   Transmembrane molecules on T and B cells with YXXL motifs in their cytoplasmic domains. Involved in receptor signal transduction pathways after tyrosine phosphyorylation.

Immunosuppressive drugs.   Drugs which inhibit any adaptive immune response.

Inflammatory response.   A response to either injury or infection which is often local. It is characterized by increased blood flow and capillary permeability, as well as diapedesis of neutrophils and macrophages out of the circulation into the inflammatory site. **Acute** inflammation can occur within minutes and usually is resorbed, but differs from **chronic** inflammation, which occurs after a persistent infection.

Innate immunity.   Nonspecific cellular and humoral first line defense. Does not increase in intensity after repeated exposure to the same or different pathogens.

Integrins. A group of heterodimeric cell-surface molecules important in cell-cell (lymphocytes and antigen presenting cells) and cell-matrix (leukocyte migration) interactions. For example, LFA-1, VLA-4, CD11b on leukocytes bind the immunoglobulin superfamily proteins, ICAMs, VCAM-1 on endothelium.

Interferons (IFN). Cytokines which help cells resist viral replication and regulate the immune response. IFNα and IFNβ (Type I) are produced primarily by leukocytes and fibroblasts and are anti-viral. IFNγ (Type II) produced by Th1 and NK cells, which can activate macrophages, upregulate MHC molecules, and promote B cells to produce IgG_{2a}.

Interleukin. A cytokine produced by leukocytes.

Intraepithelial lymphocytes (IEL). Found between epithelial cells lining mucosal surfaces. Part of the mucosal-associated lymphoid tissue defense system. Mainly $CD8^+$ T cells, 10-40% of which are TCRγδ. Produce IFNγ and IL5. Function in immune surveillance with reactivity to bacterial 60-65kDa heat shock proteins.

Intron. The intervening sequences of nucleotides between exons that encode protein.

Invariant chain. Binds to MHC II molecules in the endoplasmic retriculum to block their ability to bind peptides. Degraded in vessicles, resulting in MHC II molecules able to bind endocytosed degraded peptides.

Isograft. Tissue transplanted between two genetically identical individuals.

Isotypes (see **Heavy chain**).

Isotype switching. During antibody production, IgM is produced first. Later, through site-specific recombination with deletion of intervening DNA in immunoglobulin heavy chain genes, IgG, IgA, and IgE are produced and secreted.

Langerhans cell. Dendritic cell with Fc receptors and found primarily in the stratum spinosum area of the epidermis. They transport antigen from the epidermis to the regional lymph node where they become interdigitating dendritic cells.

Large granular lymphocytes (LGLs). A group of morphologically defined lymphocytes which include NK cells.

Leukocyte. All white blood cells, including lymphocytes, polymorphonuclear leukocytes, and monocytes.

Leukotrienes. Metabolic products of arachidonic acid that serve as lipid mediators of inflammation. Also called slow reacting substance of anaphylaxis (SRS-A).

Light chain. Smaller of the two chains of an antibody molecule. Has a variable domain (V_L) and a constant domain (C_L). Two types, κ and λ.

L-selectin. Adhesion molecule on lymphocytes that binds CD34 and Gly-CAM-1 on high endothelial venules to initiate lymphocyte diapedesis.

Lymph nodes. Important secondary lymphoid organs with a blood supply and receiving afferent lymphatic vessels. Cells that leave the parenchyma exit via efferent lymphatics to the thoracic duct.

Lymphopoiesis. Differentiation and generation of lymphocytes from hematopoietic stem cells.

Lymphotoxin (TNFβ, LTα). Cytokine produced by leukocytes, primarily $CD4^+$ cells, which can cause necrosis. Important in normal secondary lymphoid tissue development, particularly in inducing follicular dendritic cell clusters.

Macrophage. Large bone marrow-derived phagocytic cells of the monocytic series, which are very important in innate immunity, and early phases of host defense. Functions also as the major antigen processing and presenting cell in adaptive immunity. Found throughout the body as the mononuclear phagocytic system. In addition, secretes IL-1, 6, 8, 10, 12, TNFα, TGFβ, GM-CSF, G-CSF, M-CSF, and functions in ADCC.

Major histocompatibility complex (MHC). Group of very polymorphic genes found on chromosome 6 in humans that encode MHC or HLA molecules. **MHC I** molecules present cytosolic peptides to CD8 T cells, **MHC II** molecules present endocytosed and lysosomal degraded peptides to CD4 T cells. Foreign surface MHC molecules function as cellular antigens and are the targets for T cells in graft rejection or GVHD.

Mantle zone. Rim of primarily resting B cells surrounding germinal centers. Also may be an exit point for cells from germinal centers.

Marginal zone and sinus. Region of spleen between red and white pulp. The zone contains B cells, memory cells and macrophages. The sinus receives cells which migrate into the white pulp.

Mast cells. Bone marrow derived cells residing in connective tissue areas similar to but different from basophils. Large granules with histamine, heparin, serotonin, chondroitin sulfate E, etc. Express Fc_ϵ receptors similar to basophils. Secrete many immunoregulatory cytokines which can effect modulation of CD4 cell polarization into Th1 or Th2 subsets.

Medulla. The central or innermost aspect of an organ with the cortex being the periphery. It is usually the collecting or exit point in an organ such as the thymus and lymph node.

Membrane attack complex (MAC). Formed at the end of the classical or alternate complement pathway and thus contain C5b-9. Mediates cell lysis by forming a transmembrane channel in the target similar to perforin.

MHC restriction. T cells will only recognize peptide if it is presented to them in the context of the MHC molecules of their maturing environment.

Microfold (M) cells. Specialized enterocytes found in primarily the ileum of the small intestine and rectum. They line the surface of Peyers patches (PP) in the ileum and are specialized in their ability to endocytose and transport antigen including viruses from the gut lumen to the underlying lymphoid tissue in the lamina propria and submucosa.

Monocytes. Bone marrow derived peripheral blood cells that are the precursors of tissue and organ macrophages and thus represent the mononuclear phagocytic system.

Mucosal associated lymphoid tissue (MALT). All **intraepithelial lymphocytes** as well as lamina propria and submucosal lymphoid tissue below mucosal lined areas. Gut associated lymphoid tissue (**GALT**) and bronchial associated lymphoid tissue (**BALT**) are components of the MALT.

Natural killer (NK) cells. A subset of large granular lymphocytes which are not T or B cells. They kill some tumor cells and virally-infected cells, as well as those cells lacking MHC I molecules but exhibit no memory. Are CD16$^+$ and CD56$^+$. Represent 5-15% of lymphocytes found in peripheral blood and spleen but as much as 25% of those found in the sinusoids of the liver where they are called **pit** cells. Do not recirculate and they are not found in the thoracic duct. Part of the innate immune system and can produce IFNγ, TNFα, and GM-CSF.

Necrosis. Extensive cell injury and death leading to debris and inflammation. In **apoptosis** there is no inflammation.

Neutrophils (neutrophilic polymorphonuclear leukocytes). The most abundant white cell in peripheral blood. Multilobed nucleus with granules that don't stain with most peripheral blood tetrachrome stains. First circulating phagocytic cell to be involved in an inflammatory response.

Nude mice. Mice which are not only hairless, but also have no thymus due to a defect in their thymic stroma and, thus, do not produce normal T cells.

Opsonization. Deposition of antibody and complement on bacteria promoting contact and destruction by phagocytic cells.

Paratope. Area in the V domain of an antibody or T cell receptor binding the **epitope** of an antigen.

Perforin. Protein, stored in the granules of cytotoxic T cells and NK cells along with **granzymes** that are released on contact with the target cell. In the presence of Ca^{++}, polymerizes to form transmembrane pores on target cells similar to those produced by the **MAC**.

Periarteriolar lymphoid sheath (PALS). Lymphocytes, primarily T cells, that surround the central arterioles which branch from trabecular arteries of the spleen. Attached to the PALS are the primary and secondary lymphoid follicles.

Phagocytosis. Internalization of a foreign particle or another cell by a phagocytic cell. Ingested material is contained in a **phagosome** which fuses with lysosomes to become a **phagolysosome**. Lysosomal enzymes degrade the material into small peptides which can occupy the MHC II groove for presentation to T or B cells.

Platelets. Small membrane bound cytoplasmic product of megakaryocytes in the bone marrow. Has granules which contain clotting factors, vasoactive substances, and growth factors (**platelet derived growth factor**).

Polymorphism. Variability at a specific gene locus. The MHC is the most polymorphic gene locus in humans.

Primary follicles.   Found in all secondary lymphoid tissue. Contain resting B cells and some follicular dendritic cells. When activated B cells (centroblasts) and Th cells enter, they become **secondary follicles** with **germinal centers**.

Primary lymphoid organs.   The bone marrow and thymus where lymphocyte precursors mature into immunocompetent antigen reactive T and B cells without having ever seen the antigen previously. These immunocompetent cells seed **secondary lymphoid organs**.

Programmed cell death   (see **Apoptosis**).

Proteosome.   A large cytosolic catalytic multisubunit protease complex that degrades cytosolic proteins to peptides for presentation by MHC I molecules.

Proto-oncogens.   Genes that encode growth-controlling proteins in normal cells.

Receptor editing.   Replacing a potentially self-reactive light chain of an antigen receptor on a developing B cell with a non-self-reactive light chain.

Recombination activating genes (RAG-1, RAG-2).   Encoding RAG-1 and RAG-2 proteins critical for variable region gene rearrangement in developing lymphocyte receptors such as the T cell receptor and B cell immunoglobulin.

Red pulp of spleen.   An area of spleen around the white pulp which contains red cells, sinusoidal macrophages, and NK cells. Site where old red cells are destroyed.

Secondary immune response.   Occurs after another exposure to antigen and involves memory cells that are activated to produce a more rapid and more pronounced response than in the **primary** response.

Selectins.   Monomeric cell-surface adhesion molecules on leukocytes (L-selectin) and endothelial cells (E- and P-selectin) that bind mucin-like CAMs on specific glycoproteins to initiate leukocyte binding to endothial interactions.

Sepsis.   Bacterial infection of the bloodstream that can trigger massive release of TNF-α and **septic shock**.

Serotonin (5-hydroxytryptamine).   Principal vasoactive amine found in basophil, mast cell, and platelet granules. Receptors on local endothelium and vascular smooth muscle.

Somatic cell hypermutation.   Point mutations introduced into rearranged imunoglobulin V-region genes during B cell activation, proliferation, and maturation. Generates variant antibodies, some of which have a higher binding affinity. Permits refinement of antibody specificity contributing to antibody diversity.

Stem cells.   Cells found in the blood islands of the yolk sac and paraaortic splanchnopleura mesenchyme of the day 7.5–8.5 embryo. Later in development, they are found in the liver, spleen, and eventually the bone marrow where they are mainly found after birth. They are $CD34^+$ and upon division their daughter cells usually give rise to a multipotential progentor cell and another stem cell.

Stroma.   The connective tissue and epithelial structural components which form the microenvironment of an organ for its **parenchyma** consisting of the circulating, sessile, and reactive cells.

Superantigens.   Certain bacterial and viral glycoproteins that bind to the

MHC II molecules on antigen presenting cells outside the peptide binding groove. They also bind to the V_β domains of the T cell receptor. The result is activation of T cells in an antigen-nonspecific and MHC-unrestricted manner.

Surface immunoglobulin. Surface membrane molecule on B cells that functions as the B cell antigen receptor.

Surrogate light chain. Two gene products V- pre-B and lamda 5 (homologous with the λIg L and V-region genes) from a light chain-like molecule. These surrogate light chains can combine with the heavy chain (IgH) protein in pro- and large pre-B cells to form a **pre-B-cell receptor**. After κ and λ L chains are synthesized, the Ig L chain displaces the surrogate from IgH so that an intact immunoglobulin is formed and delivered to the cell surface.

Syngeneic. A graft of tissue or cells between two genetically identical individuals.

TAP-1 and TAP-2 (transporters associated with antigen processing). Transporters of short peptides from the cytosol to the endoplasmic reticulum lumen where the short peptides bind MHC I molecules. Required for proper expression of MHC I molecules.

T cell receptor. A disulfide-linked heterodimer on the surface of T cells complexed with the CD3 chains. Most receptors on peripheral T cells are highly variable $\alpha\beta$ dimers, but some are $\gamma\delta$ at musosal epithelial surfaces.

Terminal deoxynucleotidyl transferase (TdT). Enzyme responsible for inserting nontemplated or N-nucleotides into junctions between gene segments in the T cell receptor or the immunoglobulin heavy chain V-region genes. These N-nucleotides contribute extensively to the diversity of V-region genes of T and B cell receptors.

Transgenic animal. Animals developed with genes placed into their original genome with specific promotors controlling their site and duration of their expression.

Tumor immunology. The immune response to tumors. Syngeneic tumors are accepted as grafts unless their MHC groove contains proteins which the host can perceive as foreign. Some tumor antigens are found on heat shock proteins.

Tyrosine kinase. Enzyme that phosphorylates the tyrosine residues of proteins, which are important in T, B, and NK cell activation. T cell has Lck, Fyn, and ZAP-70. B cell has Blk, Fyn, Lyn, and Syk.

V (variable) gene segment. Represented by the $5'$ coding portion of rearranged B-cell immunoglobulin and T-cell receptor genes. When one of many potential V-gene segments rearranges to a J or DJ segment, an intact V-domain exon is produced which pairs with a different V region to form the complete receptor.

White pulp. The lymphoid tissue area of the spleen separated from the **red pulp** by the marginal zone and sinus. That part surrounding the central artery called the periarteriolar lymphoid sheath (**PALS**) which contain primarily T cells.

Xenogeneic. Belonging to individuals of another species.

Xenograft. Transplants of tissue or cells between species.

· A P P E N D I X · 1 ·

CD ANTIGENS

CD	CELLULAR EXPRESSION	FUNCTIONS
1a,b,c	Cortical Thymocytes, B cells, Langerhans and Dendritic Cells	MHC-I like, associated with β_2-microglobulin. Role in lipid Ag presentation.
2 (LFA-2)	T and NK cells	Adhesion molecule binds to CD58 (LFA-3). Associated with intracellular Lck.
3 ($\gamma\epsilon, \delta\epsilon$, $\zeta\zeta$ or $\zeta\eta$)	Thymocytes, T cells	Associated with the surface T cell receptor (TCR) and required for TCR signal transduction. ζ and η also associated with surface TCR but have cytoplasmic domains with ITAM motifs that bind to cytoplasmic tyrosine kinases.
4	Subset of thymocytes, Th1, Th2, monocytes	Associative recognition element or co-receptor for TCR. Associated with Lck. Receptor for gp 120 on HIV.
8	Subset of thymocytes, CTL	Associative recognition element or co-receptor for TCR. Associated with Lck.
11a (LFA-1)	Leukocytes	Adhesion molecule associated with CD18. Binds to CD54 (ICAM-1), ICAM-2, and ICAM-3
11b (Mac-I/ CR3)	Myeloid and NK cells	Associated with CD18. Binds iC3b, ICAM-1, and fibrinogen.
11c (CR4)	Myeloid Cells	Associated with CD18. Binds fibrinogen.
16	Phagocytes, NK cells	FcγR III component. Necessary for ADCC and phagocytosis.
18	Leukocytes	Integrin B_2. Associates with CD11a, b, and c.
19	B cells	Complexes with CD21 (CR2). Co-receptor for B cell activation as cytoplasmically binds tyrosine and PI-3 kinases.
21	B cells, FDC	Complexes with CD19 and 21 to form co-receptor for B cell activation. Binds iC3b and E-B virus.

(continued)

CD ANTIGENS *(continued)*

CD	CELLULAR EXPRESSION	FUNCTIONS
25	Activated T and B cells, monocytes	IL-2 receptor
28	T and activated B cells	Co-stimulatory signaling. Binds CD80 (B7.1) and B7.2 (CD86).
29	Leukocytes	Adhesion molecule.
34	Hematopoietic stem cells	Ligand for CD62L (L selectin).
35 (CR1)	Erythrocytes, phagocytic cells FDC, B cells	Binds to C3b and C4b. Mediates phagocytosis.
40	B cells, macrophages, dendritic cells, thymic epithelial cells (TEC)	Binds to CD40 Ligand (L), receptor for co-stimulatory signal for B cell growth, differentiation, and isotype switching. Promotes cytokine production by macrophages, dendritic, and TEC.
40L	Activated CD4 cells	Ligand for CD40
45	All lymphocytes	A tyrosine phosphatase used in B and T cell signaling. Multiple isoforms.
45RA (B220)	B cells, naive T cells	CD45 isoform with A exon
54 (ICAM-1)	Leukocytes and non-hematopoietic cells	Adhesion molecule that binds LFA-1 and Mac-1
55 (DAF)	Hematopoietic and nonhematopoietic cells	Binds C3b
58 (LFA-3)	Hematopoietic and nonhematopoietic cells	Binds CD2
59 (Protectin)	Hematopoietic and nonhematopoietic cells	Binds C8 and C9 to block MAC assembly
80 (B7.1)	B cells, macrophages, dendritic cells	Ligand for CD28 and CTLA-4 co-stimulatory molecule
86 (B7.2)	B cells, macrophages dendritic cells	Ligand for CD28 and CTLA-4 co-stimulatory molecule
95 (FAS)	Wide cellular distribution	Binds to FAS-Ligand (FAS-L) and induces apoptosis

IMPORTANT CYTOKINES

CYTOKINES	MAJOR SOURCE	MAIN ACTIONS	ACTIONS ANTAGONIZED BY
IL-1	M/M, Epithelia[a]	Proinflammatory[b] acute phase protein production	Il-1 RA
IL-2	Th1	Th1 and B cell growth	anti-CD25
IL-3	T cells, TEC	Multilineage stem cell growth	?
IL-4	Th2, mast cells, basophils	Stimulates B and Th2. Stimulates IgG_4 and IgE switch.	IFN-γ
IL-5	Th2	Growth of eosinophils and B cells	IFN-γ
IL-6	M/M, Th2	B, T, NK cell growth. Proinflammatory. Acute phase protein production.	?
IL-7	Marrow stromal and TEC	Growth of late pro-B/ early pre-B, and immature thymocytes	?
IL-8	M/M, TEC	Proinflammatory. Neutrophil chemotactic.	?
IL-10	M/M, some T cells	Potent down regulator of M/M function and Th1 responses.	INF-γ
IL-12	M/M, B cells	Critical activator of NK responsiveness and Th1 development	IL-10
IL-13	Th2	B cell growth. Anti-proinflammatory.	IFN-γ
Interferon (IFN) α, β (Type I)	Leukocytes, fibroblasts	Anti-viral. Increased MHC-I expression.	Unknown
IFN-γ	Th1, NK cells	M/M activator.	IL-10, 4

(continued)

[a] Monocytes/Macrophages.

[b] Macrophage activation, fever, T cell activation.

IMPORTANT CYTOKINES *(continued)*

CYTOKINES	MAJOR SOURCE	MAIN ACTIONS	ACTIONS ANTAGONIZED BY
(Type II)		Up regulator MHCI/II. Promotes B cell→IgG$_{2a}$ production.	
TNF-α (cachectin)	M/M, NK cells activated T cells	Proinflammatory. Primary mediator of systemic infection Apoptosis. Upregulated MHC-I. Promotes normal secondary lymphoid tissue development.	IL-10
TNF-β (lymphotoxin; LTα)	Leukocytes	Cell death. Sepsis Promotes normal secondary lymphoid tissue development.	?
TGF-β	M/M, T cells chondrocytes, TEC	Down regulates Th1. Anti-inflammatory.	?
MIF	T cells	Inhibits macrophage migration	?
CD40L	Th	B cell activation. Class switching.	?
FAS-L	Activated T cells	Apoptosis	?
GM-CSF	M/M, T cells, TEC	Growth and differentiation of myelomonocytic cells	?
G-CSF	Fibroblasts, TEC, M/M, endothelial cells	Neutrophil development	?
M-CSF (CSF-1)	Stromal cells, fibroblasts, TEC, endothelial, M/M	M/M development.	?
Epo (Erythropoietin)	Kidney cortex	Stimulates erythroid progenitors	?
Thrombopoietin	Kidney, liver, bone marrow, spleen	Stimulates magakaryo-poiesis and erythroid progenitors	?

• I N D E X •

Locators for tables and figures are enclosed in brackets [ ].

Accessory molecules
CD3-T cell receptor (TCR) complex,
87, [88]
Acquired immunity. *See* Adaptive
immunity
Acute inflammatory response
role in nonspecific immunity, 149, 150
Adaptive immunity
cells central to response, [3], 3–4
defined, 2
innate immunity vs., 2
Adhesion
mediation by lymphocyte integrin proteins, 111
Adhesion molecules. *See also* Cell adhesion molecules
role in exits and entries with vascular
distribution system, 134
Adjuvants
role in antigen immunogenic potential,
25–26
Adrenocorticotropin hormone (ACTH)
role in endocrine-immune autoregulatory loop, 180, 181
role in immune cell function, 184
Ag
B cell presentation, 112
cell traffic in gut, [115]
Aged
neuroendocrine-immune autoregulatory loop effects, 183
Allelic exclusion
B cell differentiation, 37
T cell differentiation, 44
Allergic response
defined, 117
eosinophils, 104
group I, 118–119
group II, 118, 119–120
group III, 118, 119–120
group IV, 118, 120
IgE-mediated
illustration, [121]
systemic anaphylaxis, 119

IgG-mediated
insoluble antigens, [122]
soluble antigens, [123]
mechanism, 117
Alloantigens
major histocompatibility complex
(MHC) role in antigen specific
immunosuppression, 177–178
Allogeneic transplants
rejection, 170
Allografts
rejection, 170
Allotypes
defined, 30
Anaphylaxis
cause, 104
group I allergic response, 118
systemic
IgE-mediated allergic response, 119
Anergy
defined, 36
Anti-inflammatory agents
effects on fibrotic process, 109
Antibodies
antigen-specific
antigen-specific T cell-dependent
antibody formation, 96
formation theories
clonal selection theory, 95–96
instructive theory, 95
network theory, 95, 96
selective theory, 95
defined, 26, 91
IgE
role in allergic response, 118
IgG
role in allergic response, 119–120
isotype production
cytokine profiles and, 99
mechanisms by which immunity is
provided, 91–92
primary and secondary responses,
93
T cell-dependent

ISBN 0-07-011371-8

CLANCY: BASIC CONCEPTS/IMM